Whiplash Injury

Andreas Otte

Whiplash Injury

New Approaches of Functional Neuroimaging

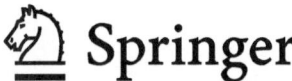 Springer

Prof. Dr. med. Andreas Otte
Faculty of Electrical Engineering
and Information Technology
Institut für Angewandte Forschung (IAF)
University of Applied Sciences Offenburg
Offenburg, Germany

ISBN 978-3-662-50855-8   ISBN 978-3-642-28356-7 (eBook)
DOI 10.1007/978-3-642-28356-7
Springer Heidelberg Dordrecht London New York

Springer is part of Springer Science+Business Media (www.springer.com)

"In bunten Bildern wenig Klarheit,
Viel Irrtum und ein Fünkchen Wahrheit".

J.W. von Goethe (1749-1832), Faust I

In motley pictures little clarity, much error and a spark of verity.

Preface

Whiplash injuries are often looked upon as accidents causing extensive symptomatology without the presence of objective findings. They can cause a disease condition, which is frequently denied, but is unfortunate and may become chronic and invalidating for the patient.

In the last two decades, much has been published on whiplash injury. However, the confusion and medicolegal discussion on this disease has increased.

In this scenario, a guide on recent and current international research in the field is even more than necessary. Especially functional imaging methods – such as single-photon emission tomography (SPET) or positron emission tomography (PET) – have shown various and sometimes differing brain alterations, which should be discussed in the conflicting arena of whiplash victims, treating physicians, insurance companies, and reviewers.

This book is a critical approach to the challenging interpretation of the aforementioned new research data of functional neuroimaging in whiplash injury. It may help patients, their relatives and friends, and involved physicians understand this condition as disease.

Offenburg, Germany

Andreas Otte

Acknowledgments

We are very happy that this book is published by one of the premier publishers in the field. This guarantees a high quality of production and allows for the inclusion of many color figures, which is an essential detail in the field of functional neuroimaging.

We would like to thank Dr. Ute Heilmann from Springer for her continuous help and input during the development of this book.

Contents

List of Abbreviations

^{11}C	Radioactive carbon-11, positron emitter
^{57}Co	Radioactive cobalt-57, gamma emitter
^{15}O	Radioactive oxygen-15, positron emitter
^{18}F	Radioactive fluorine-18, positron emitter
^{99m}Tc	Radioactive technetium-99m, gamma emitter
AC-PC line	Line between anterior and posterior commissure of the brain
CT	Computer(ized) tomography
ECD	^{99m}Tc ECD (ethylene biyldicysteinate dimer, Neurolite™), perfusion marker used in SPET
EEG	Electroencephalography
FDG	Fluorodeoxy-D-glucose, glucose analogon; labeled with the positron emitter fluorine-18, it is used in PET as glucose metabolism marker
fMRI	Functional magnetic resonance imaging
g	Acceleration constant of the earth
GMI	Glucose metabolic index
HMPAO	^{99m}Tc HMPAO (hexamethyl propylene amine oxime, Ceretec™), perfusion marker used in SPET
MEG	Magnetoencephalography
MR/PET	Combination of magnetic resonance imaging and positron emission tomography in a hybrid scanner system
MRI	Magnetic resonance imaging
ms	Millisecond
NK1	(Substance P) neurokinin-1, receptor
PET	Positron emission tomography
PET/CT	Combination of positron emission tomography and computer tomography in a hybrid scanner system
PI	Perfusion index
ROI	Region of interest
rCBF	Regional cerebral blood flow
SPET	Single-photon emission tomography
SPET/CT	Combination of single-photon emission tomography and computer tomography in a hybrid scanner system
SQUID	Superconducting quantum interference device
Δv	Change of speed

Introduction

"Arma virumque cano, Troiae qui primus ab oris
Italiam fato profugus Lavinaque venit
litora – multum ille et terris iactatus et alto
vi superum, saevae memorem Iunonis ob iram,
multa quoque et bello passus, dum conderet urbem
inferretque deos Latio – genus unde Latinum
Albanique patres atque alta moenia Romae."[1]

- Publius Vergilius Maro (70–19 B.C.), Aeneïs

1.1 General Aspects

Whiplash injury (with a distortion of the cervical spine) and its consequence
(the late whiplash syndrome) are a continuously controversial medicolegal challenge. The ongoing ambiguity with the presence and extent of the late whiplash
syndrome leads to multiple disconcertion not only in the accident victims but also
in treating physicians, attorneys, judges, or insurance companies.

1.1.1 The Term "Whiplash Injury"

By definition, no head impact may be associated with a whiplash injury. Since the
introduction of head restraints into the modern automobile this, however, in most
cases does not apply any more. Collision forces, which do not have to necessarily
leave traces, can lead to so-called closed head injuries. Even with a pure acceleration mechanism without head impact, it can come to direct cerebral injuries
(Fig. 1.1), as *Ommaya and coworkers* could show already in 1968 in a monkey
experiment (Ommaya et al. 1968).

---

[1] "I sing of arms and the man, who – exiled by fate – first came from the Trojan coasts to Italy and
the Lavine shores; was much smitten on land and sea by violence from Heaven, through cruel Juno's
unforgiving wrath, and suffered much in war, until he could found the city and bring over his gods
to Latium, from where arose the Latin race, the fathers of Alba and the high walls of Rome."

A. Otte, *Whiplash Injury*,
DOI 10.1007/978-3-642-28356-7_1, © Springer-Verlag Berlin Heidelberg 2012

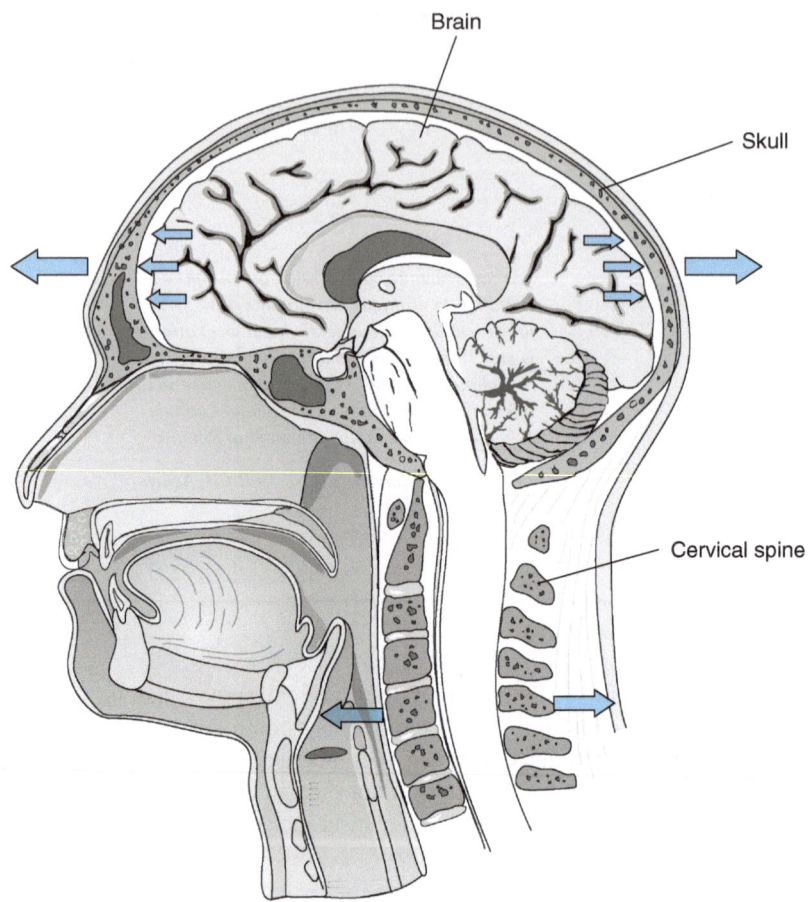

Fig. 1.1 "Whiplash" injury: In whiplash injury, apart from the cervical spine, also the head, which is embodied at it, moves. In the head, the brain can be likewise pulled by impact on the bone wall (Adapted from Otte et al. (eds) (2004) Nuclear Medicine in Psychiatry, Springer, Heidelberg)

1.1.2 Symptoms

In all stages of a whiplash injury by acceleration forces, in addition to peripheral symptoms such as neck pain and neck rigidity, it can come to central, i.e., cerebral, symptoms. According to the *Quebec Task Force on Whiplash Associated Disorders* (Spitzer et al. 1995), these cerebral symptoms comprise headache, dizziness, vertigo, tinnitus, concentration, attention and memory disturbances, and temporomandibular dysfunction. Furthermore, often visual symptoms such as blurred vision or oscillopsia are reported.

Both the peripheral as well as the central symptoms arise typically with a characteristic latency of 0–72 h. Especially the cerebral symptoms are of utmost relevance

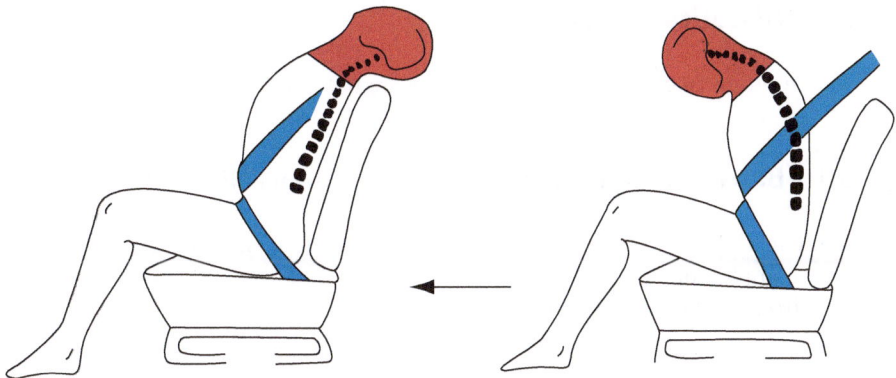

Fig. 1.2 Scheme of a typical whiplash mechanism, e.g., following a rear-end car collision. During sudden acceleration of the fixed trunk, the unfixed head is accelerated first to the rear and then forward. Already low speeds between 10 and 20 km/h can cause large acceleration forces on the head (Croft 1998; Olsson et al. 1990; Ryan et al. 1993) (Adapted from Otte et al. (eds) (2004) Nuclear Medicine in Psychiatry, Springer, Heidelberg)

for the development of chronic stages and often subject to the various controversial discussions on the causality of the disease. The frequent absence of objective findings in the late whiplash syndrome increases this problem.

In this situation, methods are welcome, which can capture the objective condition of the brain. Due to the controversial discussion of the topic, such methods are, however, often rejected.

1.2 Incidence

Whiplash injuries may occur anywhere: in traffic accidents, accidents at sports, or at work. They are not necessarily limited to car accidents with a rear-end collision mechanism, although rear-end car collisions represent the most frequent cause for whiplash trauma. Crucial is only the accident mechanism, i.e., the presence of a cervical distortion with or without cerebral participation (Fig. 1.2).

According to the *Quebec Task Force on Whiplash Associated Disorders* (Spitzer et al. 1995), only about 5% of the whiplash-injured develop a chronic disease beyond 1 year after the accident.

According to Schmid (1999), the incidence of whiplash injuries in the industrialized countries is up to 3.8 cases per 1,000 inhabitants per year. Evans (1992) reported of more than one million cases per year in the United States. A careful estimation of the general federation of the German insurance economy in Munich calculated about 0.5 to 1 billion € of subsequent annual costs in Germany. Within the European Union, the subsequent costs are estimated at least 10 billion € per year. The largest portion of these costs comprises substitution of the failing regular income.

1.3   Historical Aspects

CNS symptoms in cervical spine alterations are not new.

1.3.1   Barré's "Syndrome Sympathique Cervical Postérieur"

Already in 1926, the French neurologist Jean Alexandre Barré described a characteristic complex of symptoms in patients with cervical diseases, which, in part, is
known from the late whiplash syndrome (Barré 1926).

1.3.2   The Term "Railway Spine"

In the nineteenth century, the (British) term "railway spine" was established in a time
where traveling by train became popular (Harrington 1996; Keller 1995; Caplan
1995; Fischer-Homberger 1970; Otte 2001a, b). It was assigned to patients with
posttraumatic symptoms and no apparent lesions after train accidents, and it was
hypothesized that these symptoms were related to molecular spinal damage. Although
the medicolegal discussion became obsolete after 1900 as a consequence of an
increasing number of malingerers and fraud, the controversy on the phenomenon
"railway spine" may have been a precursor for some of the discussion on posttraumatic symptoms today.

1.3.3   Maurice Ravel

Maurice Ravel (1875–1937), the French impressionistic and, in his later years, clas-
sicistic composer, had a taxi accident in 1932, where he lost a few of his teeth and
suffered from a short mild concussion. It is reported that he was treated by "needles"
and hypnosis (Otte et al. 2003a, b; Otte and Wink 2008). The usual interpretation of
Ravel's symptoms during his disease is Pick's disease with primary progressive apha-
sia (Otte et al. 2003b). Linked to the taxi accident in 1932, Ravel, however, developed additional deficits in concentration and attention and lost his ability to complete
any new composition (Table 1.1). Also his appearance deteriorated dramatically after
this accident within only a few years (Fig. 1.3a, b). The question of whether Maurice
Ravel had a distortion of the cervical spine resulting from acceleration forces and a
consecutive late whiplash syndrome or a mild to moderate brain injury, of course,
cannot be answered today. These diseases were not even known or defined at that
time. Besides, functional imaging modalities were not available, and X-ray modalities, although discovered already in 1895, were still at the beginning of their development and some years away from the development of the first computerized tomography
(CT) scanner by Godfrey Hounsfield, which first was commercially available from
the British company Electric and Musical Industries (EMI) in 1972. Nevertheless,
there seem to be interesting parallels between the symptoms subsequent to Ravel's

Table 1.1 Table comparing Ravel's major compositions with his major life events. After the taxi accident in 1932, Ravel was not able to write down any new composition, although his head was full of ideas

Compositions		Events
	1875	Birth
	1889	Music student at the Conservatoire of Music in Paris (1889–1905)
Habanera	1895	
Shéhérazade	1898	
Pavane pour une infante défunte (piano)	1899	
Jeux d'eaux	1901	
3 Shéhérazade Songs	1903	
Miroirs	1905	
Histoires naturelles	1906	
Rhapsodie espagnole; Gaspard de la nuit	1908	Death of father
Pavane pour une infante défunte (orchestra)	1910	
L'heure espagnole; Valses nobles et sentimentales	1911	
Ballet Daphnis et Chloé	1912	
Piano trio	1914	
Tombeau de Couperin (piano)	1917	Death of mother
Tombeau de Couperin (orchestra)	1919	Health cure in Mégève (fever, pulse alterations, insomnia, senile involution)
La Valse	1920	
	1921	Bought his country house near Paris
Mussorgskij: Tableaux d'une exposition (orchestration)	1922	
Tzigane	1924	
Opera "L'enfant et les sortilèges"	1925	
Chansons madécasses	1926	
	1927	Difficulties in playing the piano, dysphasia, beginning apraxia
Boléro	1928	*Doctor honoris causa* (Oxford University)
2 piano concertos	1929	
(D major for the left hand; G major for both hands)	1930	
3 chansons Don Quichotte à Dulcinée	1932	Taxi accident; aphasia, agraphia, apraxia, and severe deficits in concentration and attention
	1934	Successless health cure at Lake of Geneva
	1935	Travel to Morocco
	1937	Neurosurgery and coma (17-Dec or 19-Dec)
		Death (28-Dec)

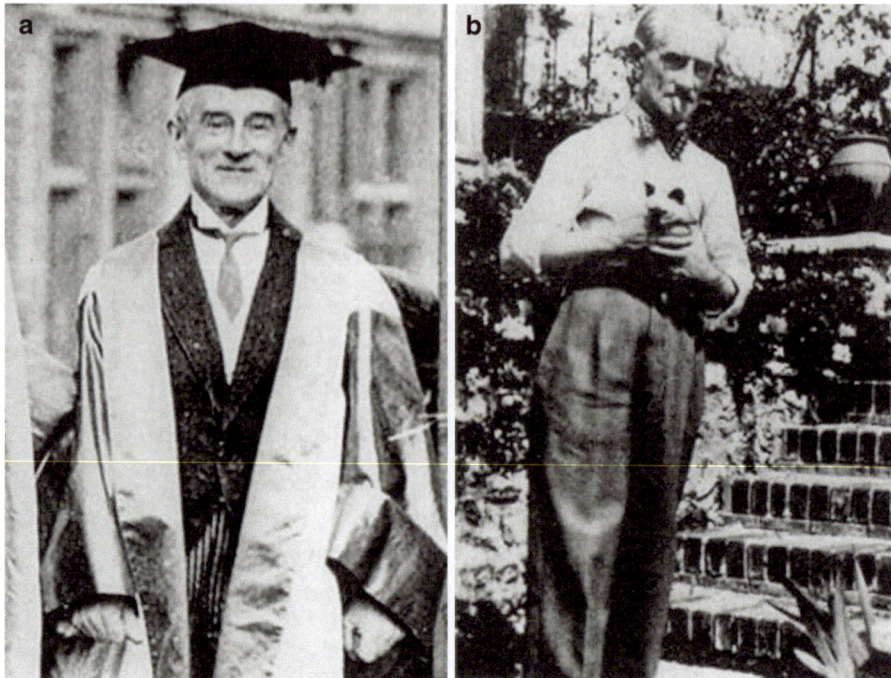

Fig. 1.3 Photographs of Maurice Ravel. (**a**) Ravel at Oxford, 1928, where he received the laureate of *doctor honoris causa*. (**b**) Ravel in his last years

taxi accident and the symptoms after whiplash injury, and we could draw this hypothetical conclusion in Ravel's case, even more as this historical case is legally unbiased today.

1.4   Biomechanics

1.4.1   General Aspects

Already in the nineteenth century, at the very beginning of the development of automobiles, people – including physicians – were about to discuss the role and dangers of acceleration forces on drivers in automobiles. The first vehicle, from Carl Benz (1844–1929), the "Patent-Motorwagen Nummer 1" from 1886 achieved a maximum speed of 16 km/h. At that time, it was assumed that this high speed would cause serious medical problems due to the high speed itself (Elis 2010).

In a detailed review from Arthur Croft, in 1998, the biomechanics in low-speed rear impact collision is described. It has not lost actuality until today. Some of the following, therefore, is derived and summarized from Croft (1998).

Already in the 1950s, first crash tests were performed. Severy et al. (1955) studied anthropometric dummies and human volunteers. In the study from Severy et al., the speed v of the car colliding with the rear end of the vehicle ahead was 16 km/h. Interestingly, the persons in the car were exposed to higher acceleration forces than the car itself: In rear-end car collisions with a Δv of 12.8 km/h, the heads of the test persons were exposed to accelerations of 5 g, whereas the car itself had an acceleration of 2 g. West et al. (1993) measured acceleration forces of the head of approximately 15 g.

Over the years, more and more crash tests were performed, and many mathematical models were developed to calculate the acceleration forces on persons in cars who were exposed to different kinds of collision mechanisms.

The forces in whiplash injury – and the according literature on this – are relatively large. The literature is also heterogeneous: Some authors described crash tests with a certain speed, and some authors a crash with an "acceleration" of a certain speed, which is not correct by definition, as an acceleration describes a change of speed (Δv) per time.

Astronauts, e.g., are accelerated to speeds of about 30,000 km/h. This is, however, not harmful, since the change in speed (Δv) is performed over a larger time.

The acceleration a is described by the following equations (Eqs. 1.1 and 1.2):

$$a = x * g; \tag{1.1}$$

and

$$x = (\Delta v)^2 / (2 * s * g) \tag{1.2}$$

with

s: length of collision

g: acceleration constant of the earth (9.80665 m/s^2)

x: (unit-less) multiplication factor ("the x-fold of g")

The following example may help to understand these equations in the car collision situation:

If we liked to determine the acceleration of the head, e.g., during a frontal collision at its contact with the windshield and we know that the windshield was moving 12.7 cm and the car moved with a speed of 40 km/h (=11.1 m/s) at collision, we can calculate x as follows (Eq. 1.2):

$$x = (11.1 \, \text{m/s})^2 / (2 * 0.127 \, \text{m} * 9.80665 \, \text{m/s}^2) = 49.5$$

This means that the acceleration in this accident situation would achieve the 49.5-fold of the acceleration constant of the earth (g). By contrast, if the head hit the rigid metal frame of the window, which only moved, e.g., 1.27 cm, the acceleration of the head would be 10 times higher, i.e., 495 g. In this case, the injury would not be survived.

The majority of rear-end car collisions are at speeds between 1 and 25 km/h, with rather minor damage on most cars. Olson et al. (1990) showed that 18% of the investigated whiplash-injured patients were exposed to rear-end car collisions with speeds <10 km/h, 60% of the patients with speeds between 10 and 20 km/h, and 22% of the patients with speeds >20 km/h. These figures could approximately be confirmed in an Australian study (Ryan et al. 1993). Interestingly, injuries due to rear-end car collisions occur more frequently with low speeds rather than with high speeds. This may be explained by the phenomenon that the collision with lower speeds is still relatively elastic, whereas the head constraints are not resistant during high Δv's. There is, however, no statistically significant correlation between the severeness of the accident and the clinical outcome.

The awareness of a collision in most cases reduces the injury grade markedly. According to Severy et al. (1955), this is caused by highly reduced forces on the head. These forces were, e.g., reduced by the car drivers by actively pushing themselves back to the seat and by activating their muscles.

In the year 1969 – the year of the landing on the moon – head restraints became mandatory for all automobiles in the USA and a few years later, in 1974, also in Germany. Head restraints help to avoid cervical injuries. Nevertheless, this protection is greatly diminished if the distance of the head from the head restraint is more than 5 cm at the beginning of the injury, as Mertz and Patrick could show already in 1967. In a study from Olsson et al. (1990) symptoms in the neck and cervical region markedly increased if the head distance from the head restraint was more than 10 cm. The majority of head restraints are, however, incorrectly positioned. In addition, there is the problem of ramping, i.e., the upward-movement of the body in the seat during a collision. Therefore, any mathematical calculations of collision sequelae are only idealized models. Reality may show much larger injury of head and neck than previously calculated.

Following the simple rules of physics, the injury grade in a rear-end car collision tends to be proportional to the size of the car hitting the front car and to negatively correlate with the size of the front car which is hit at its rear end.

1.4.2   Protection Systems to Avoid Whiplash Injury

Over the past years, various automobile industries have developed protection systems against whiplash injury, which diminish the acceleration forces on the neck and the spine occurring already in rear-end car collisions with relatively low speeds. These systems are, e.g., "WHIPS," the "active head restraint," shock-resistant bumper systems, or the rear-end car collision assistance systems with radar sensors, which activate seat belts and position the head restraints correctly.

Although air bags (in the steering wheel) are not activated during pure rear-end car collisions, many of the patients with cervical spine injury have been involved in accidents with activation of the air bag. The air bag can have positive and negative implications on whiplash injury; its usefulness in terms of the whiplash syndrome is, however, controversially discussed. There are also commercially available head restraints with self-inflating air bag systems.

The impact of all of these new protection systems on the severity of the accident cases needs further investigation.

1.4.3 Sequence of Phases During a Typical Whiplash Injury

After this general introduction in biomechanical processes in rear-end car collisions, we would now like to discuss the sequence of phases during a typical whiplash injury.

Two of the important contributions to understanding this sequence of phases during whiplash injury, which is caused by low speeds, are from McConnell et al. (1993, 1995). The group investigated healthy adult men in unbraked crash tests with Δv's of <3.2 km/h till 10.9 km/h. Cars with different weight were used, and the healthy volunteers undertook different tests during several days. Some of the volunteers complained about intermittent neck pain or other symptoms due to the tests, whereas none developed long-term complaints. The collision tests and the complex acceleration and deceleration processes during the collisions were recorded on high-speed films. In the first study from 1993, an exemplary test at 7.8 km/h speed recorded the following sequence of whiplash phases (Fig. 1.4):

1. *Initial phase* (0–100 ms): The crashed car moved beneath the test person compressing the seat back cushion. At first, this caused a movement of the hips and the low back to the front, whereas at the same time, the upper part of the seat back cushion began a flexion to the rear end due to the weight of the torso.
2. *Principal forward acceleration* (100–200 ms): In this phase, the seat back cushion achieved its maximum flexion to the rear end of approximately 10°, as compared to the initial position. The volunteer moved to the upper front, and the cervical region was extended axially to the upper rear end. At the same time, the head rotated to the rear end. At 160 ms, the vertical movement of the torso started to pull the neck to the front, while the head continued to move into extension position.
3. *Torso recovery/head overspeed* (relatively higher speed of the head compared to the torso; 200–300 ms): At 200 ms, the maximum extension of head and neck and the maximum vertical movement were achieved. At 250 ms, the head began its forward movement and the torso moved downwards along the seat back cushion, while the seat back cushion had moved back to its initial position.
4. *Head deceleration/torso rest* (300–400 ms): In this phase, the declination of the head was complete and the torso was moving with the car speed. At the end of this phase, the active deceleration by intended intervention of the volunteer was achieved. The head of the volunteer gradually moved back into its initial position.
5. *Restitution phase* (400–600 ms): At 450 ms, all body parts were moving with the car speed. Movements from the collision were nearly finished.

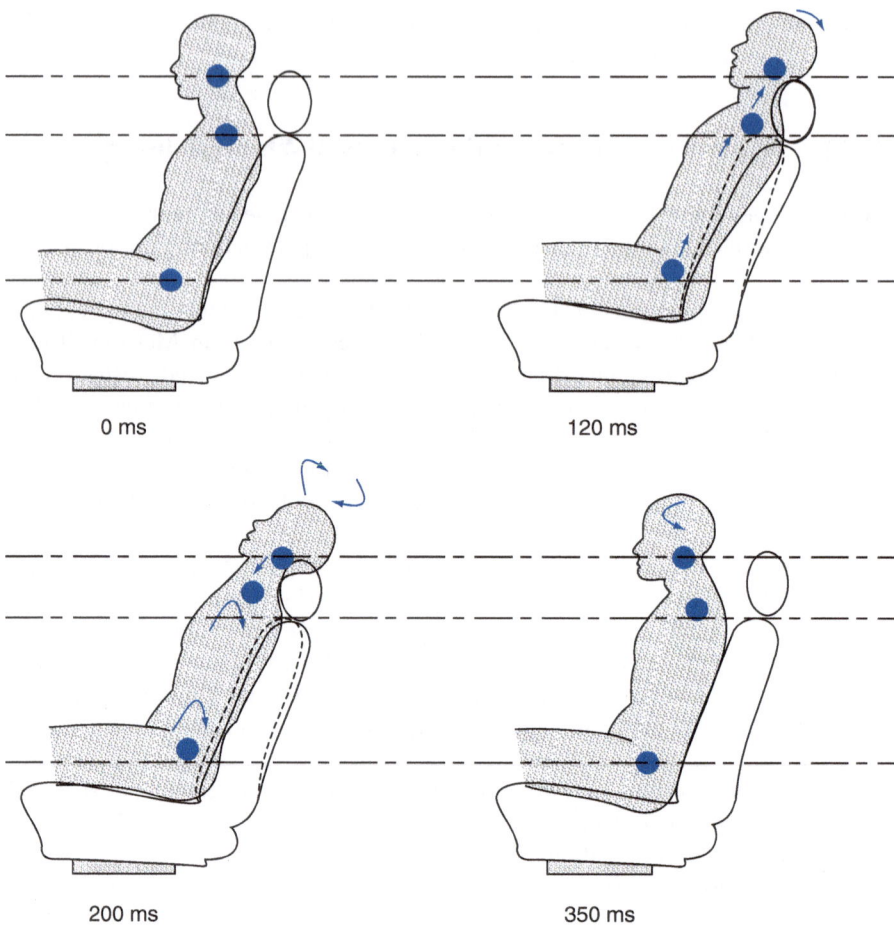

0 ms   120 ms

200 ms   350 ms

Fig. 1.4 Sequence of phases in whiplash injury (Modified from McConnell et al. (1993). (Adapted from Otte (2001) Das Halswirbelsäulen-Schleudertrauma: Neue Wege der funktionellen Bildgebung des Gehirns - Ein Ratgeber für Ärzte und Betroffene, Springer, Heidelberg) For details, see text)

Although this fascinating study for the first time revealed the dynamics of whiplash injury relatively precisely, the following potential pitfalls must certainly be realized:

- Brakes were not used.
- Volunteers tried to be correctly in position.
- Volunteers were aware of the collision.
- Only healthy men, no females or children, were included.

Diagnostics

2

2.1 Diagnostic Procedure After Whiplash Injury

The usual diagnostic procedure in whiplash injury is illustrated in Fig. 2.1.

Unfortunately, methods assessing the condition of the brain are frequently not utilized. These methods are:

1. Computerized tomography (CT) and magnetic resonance imaging (MRI) of the brain: With these methods usually no pathological cerebral findings are found in whiplash injury.
2. Neuropsychological tests: The role of neuropsychological tests for this indication is at present still being discussed.
3. Functional neuroimaging: Functional neuroimaging devices are quite sensitive measuring instruments, which are of help in the puzzling diagnosis of the late whiplash syndrome subsequent to a whiplash injury. Especially functional neuroimaging using the nuclear medicine devices single-photon emission tomography (SPET) or positron emission tomography (PET) in combination with stereotaxic brain slice delineation (e.g., Talairach and Tournoux 1988, 1993) and statistical parametric and nonparametric mapping (SPM) software developed by Friston et al. (1991, 1995a, b) is currently of essential value. In addition, functional MRI, magnetic resonance spectroscopy, superconducting quantum interference device (SQUID) magnetoencephalography (MEG), and the new hybrid imaging technologies – such as PET/CT, SPET/CT, or MR/PET – may be future methods of functional neuroimaging interest in this indication. Due to the rapid change in the development of functional neuroimaging devices, we have excluded a detailed description of these from this book. A currently detailed and state-of-the-art review on these – including image analysis tools – can, e.g., be found in Otte and Halsband (2006).
4. Other imaging devices, such as electroencephalography (EEG) or near-infrared (nIR) spectroscopy, are important diagnostic procedures in neurosciences, but have not yet been helpful in the diagnostics of whiplash patients due to their limited spatial resolution. In these devices, future developments of medical engineering industry would be most favorable.

A. Otte, *Whiplash Injury*,
DOI 10.1007/978-3-642-28356-7_2, © Springer-Verlag Berlin Heidelberg 2012

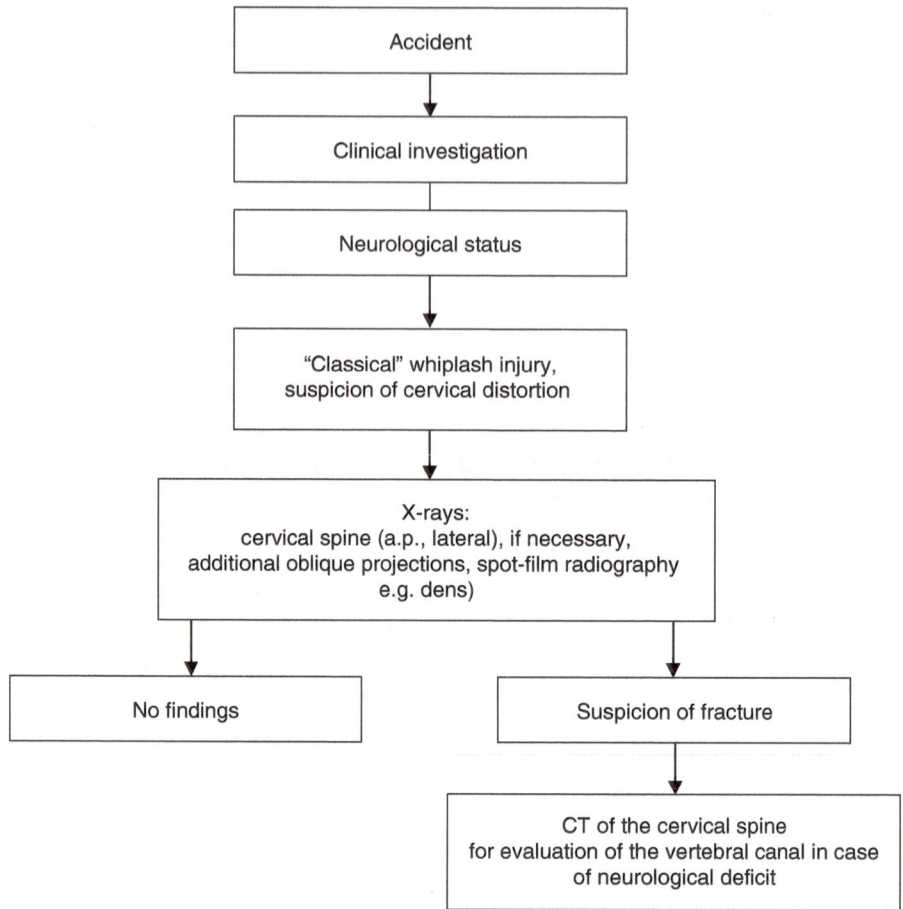

Fig 2.1 Usual diagnostic procedure in whiplash injury. Imaging of the brain is routinely not performed (Strongly modified from Jörg and Menger (1998), Schmid (1999), adapted from Otte et al. (eds) (2004) Nuclear Medicine in Psychiatry, Springer, Heidelberg)

2.2   New Iteration Algorithms

Over the last 10 years, software technologies have helped to create iteration algorithms for SPET, which convincingly improve the signal-to-noise ratio of reconstructed images. These new iteration algorithms, such as ordered subset expectation maximization (OSEM) or depth response ordered subsets expectation maximization (DROSEM), have meanwhile replaced the conventional filtered back projection. Perfusion studies with ^{99m}Tc-labeled ethylene biyldicysteinate dimer, Neurolite™ (ECD) or hexamethyl propylene amine oxime, Ceretec™ (HMPAO SPET) have become attractive and cheap in the clinical routine. For the diagnostics of potential functional alterations in whiplash injury, they are as recommendable as glucose

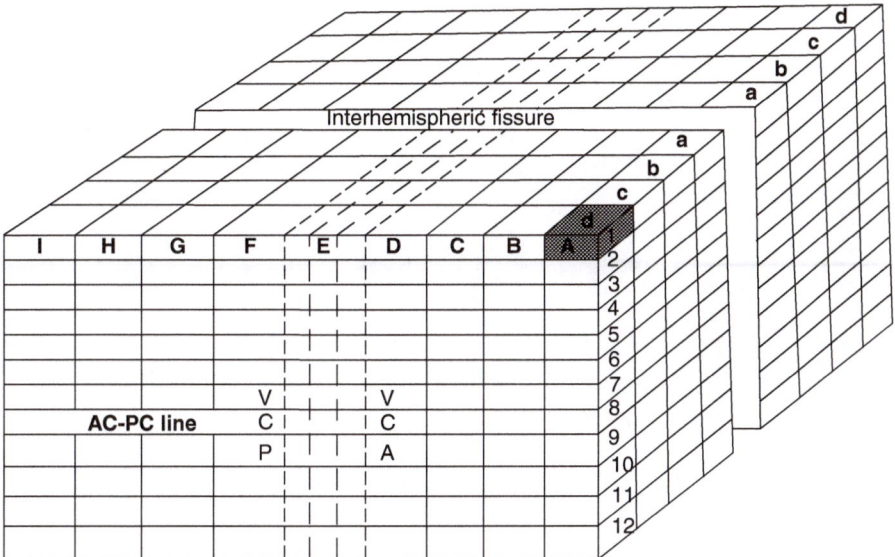

Fig. 2.2 Talairach and Tournoux atlas 3D grid for the brain from 1988. AC-PC line: line between anterior and posterior commissure of the brain. The brain is "pressed" into this volume box, accurately enabling to define the coordinates of each voxel on a standardized basis (Adapted from Otte (2001) Das Halswirbelsäulen-Schleudertrauma: Neue Wege der funktionellen Bildgebung des Gehirns - Ein Ratgeber für Ärzte und Betroffene, Springer, Heidelberg)

utilization studies by Fluorodeoxy-D-glucose, glucose analogon; labeled with the positron emitter fluorine-18, it is used in PET as glucose metabolism marker (^{18}F-FDG PET).

2.3   Stereotaxic Atlas of Talairach and Tournoux

The basis for SPM analysis of brain alterations is the coordinate system according to Talairach and Tournoux. We would, therefore, like to describe this atlas and the idea behind it in more detail.

Talairach and coworkers had already finished an atlas for the basal ganglia of the human brain in 1958. The first edition of the whole brain was published in 1967 entitled *Atlas d´Anatomie Stéréotaxique du Télencéphale*.

In this atlas, a new idea was proposed: a proportional stereotaxic grid showing the anatomy of the brain in a standardized coordinate system. For this atlas, Talairach studied in total 20 full brains and 100 hemispheres, which he compared with 400 neuroradiological assessments. For the anatomical sections, the AC-PC line (line between anterior and posterior commissure) determined by the neuroradiological image data was taken as the reference line and anatomical slices were cut in parallel to this line. From this, a 3D grid was created, which is defined by three main lines and 6 reference voxels (Fig. 2.2).

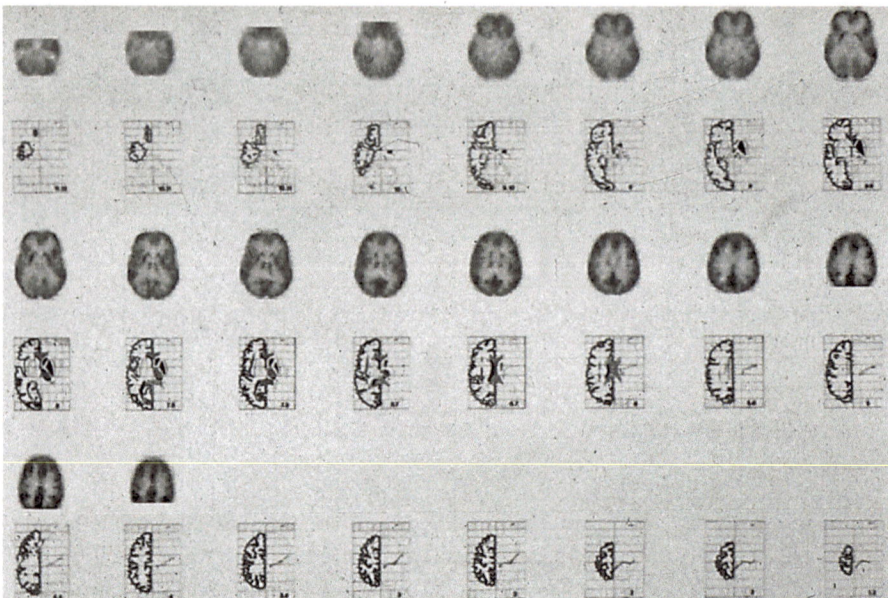

Fig. 2.3 Example from the *Talairach and Tournoux* atlas. Transversal slices from the digitized atlas are exhibited with the corresponding PET slices, which are normalized according to the *Talairach* atlas (Modified from Otte (2001) Das Halswirbelsäulen-Schleudertrauma: Neue Wege der funktionellen Bildgebung des Gehirns - Ein Ratgeber für Ärzte und Betroffene, Springer, Heidelberg)

According to this coordinate system, the Talairach reference brain was defined.

The Talairach atlas shows all brain slices of the three dimensions of the Talairach coordinate system. In its version from 1988, it has become a European standard. In the first edition (1967), the atlas was produced from six brains of different sizes in order to demonstrate the validity of the stereotaxic coordinate system. This atlas comprised 32 sagittal slices from the hemispheres of two brains, 22 and 24 coronal slices from two further brains, and each 18 transversal slices from a third pair of brains. By contrast, in the 1988 version of the Talairach atlas, only one brain of a mid-European woman is taken as the anatomical reference. In Fig. 2.3, an example from the Talairach atlas is shown along with the corresponding PET slices in transversal projection.

2.4   Statistical Parametric Mapping (SPM)

Over now nearly two decades, the freely available software package from the Wellcome Department of Cognitive Neurology, London, known as SPM (versions SPM'94 up to SPM'99, and SPM2 up to SPM8, which are all based on SPM'94 and use MATLAB (The MathWorks, Inc.) functions and subroutines), has helped in the standardization of measurement and data analysis in

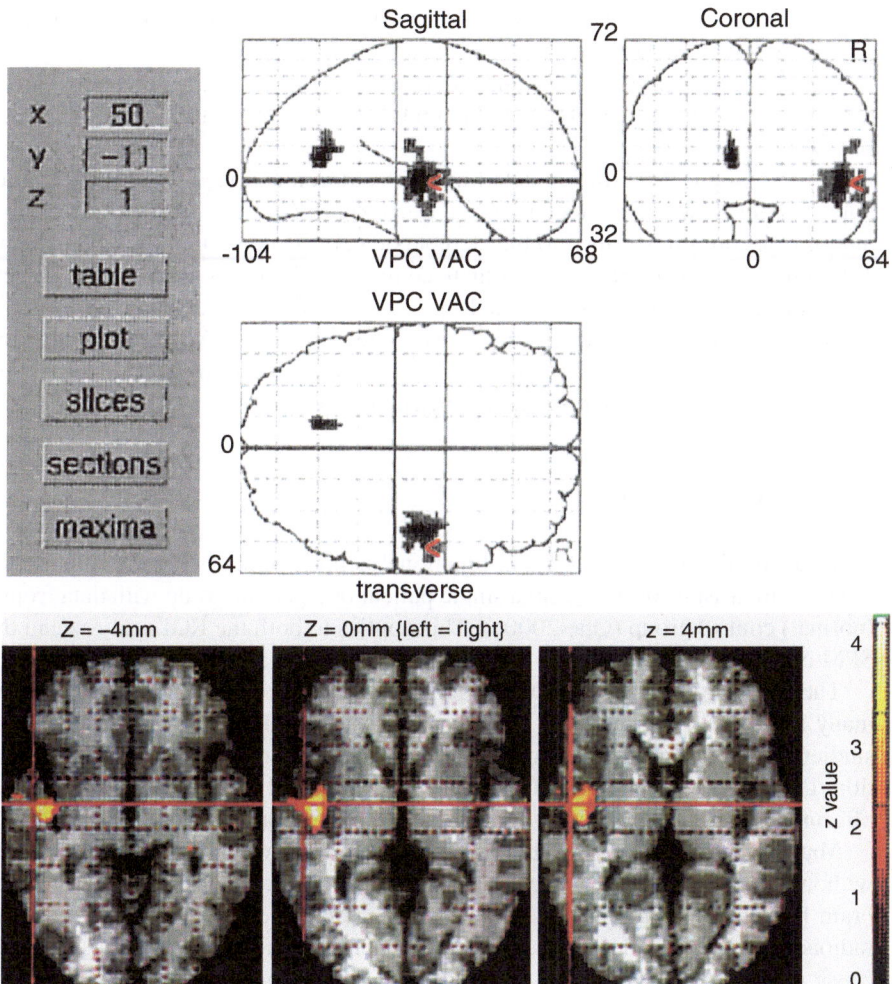

Fig. 2.4 Example of statistical parametric mapping (SPM) used in PET (Adapted from Otte (2001) Das Halswirbelsäulen-Schleudertrauma: Neue Wege der funktionellen Bildgebung des Gehirns - Ein Ratgeber für Ärzte und Betroffene, Springer, Heidelberg)

functional neuroimaging comprising analysis of fMRI, PET, SPET, EEG, and MEG data. Generally, its idea is based on the region-of-interest (ROI) technique with the difference that the regions-of-interest are now voxels in a standardized stereotaxic room. This software not only spatially normalizes PET, SPET, or fMRI images to the standardized stereotaxic Talairach and Tournoux atlas (1988) but it can also perform statistical analyses on study groups on a voxel-by-voxel basis (Friston et al. 1991, 1995a, b); this allows for reliable and objective image handling that could improve interstudy variability due to the analytical process itself. An example of SPM used in PET taken from Otte (2001c) is given in Fig. 2.4.

The various versions of SPM and a detailed description of the procedure can be retrieved from the following internet homepage for free: http://www.fil.ion.ucl. ac.uk/spm/

This method is described in detail under the aforementioned link. In brief, after interfile conversion of the reconstructed transaxial brain files into ANALYZE format, images are transformed to the stereotaxic coordinate system of Talairach and Tournoux using SPM. Then, the normalized images of patients and healthy subjects are compared by computing a voxel-by-voxel t-statistic. The t-statistic is transformed to a normal statistic yielding a Z score for each voxel. Voxels exceeding the significance level are then displayed in a "glass view" of transverse, sagittal, and coronal projections of a statistical parametric mapping.

2.5   Control Group

Any quantitative image analysis in functional neuroimaging is based on interindividual comparisons of data from a single patient or a patient group with data from a (normal) control group (Otte 2000c). This applies to both the ROI analysis and the SPM method (Friston et al. 1991, 1995a, b).

The recruitment of healthy volunteers is rather easy in some countries, but in many European countries, it is difficult, as most ethical committees do not allow studies with exposition of radioactivity to healthy volunteers without any indication. If they do so, then it is only under strict regulation. Besides, the payment and offering of incentives to healthy volunteers has become a contentious issue today.

Many institutions try to resolve this challenge by allowing for data from patients without brain alterations on previous scans or from oncological cases outside the brain having an additional ("normal") brain scan without the need for a further radioactive injection. However, especially in functional neuroimaging, this can cause potential pitfalls: Firstly, such additional scans often follow other methodological protocols as compared with standardized brain scans; secondly, oncological patients may have brain alterations (e.g., Tashiro et al. 2000). Taking such oncological patients as a "normal control group" is, therefore, dangerous and may cause conflicting challenges in the evaluation of brain lesions not only in patients who are involved in compensation cases.

It is, of course, permissible to choose a group of patients with a known brain disease as a differential diagnostic control group. Furthermore, it is important to match the control group in age and gender and to perform a substantiated statistical power calculation for the number of control subjects needed.

Hence, caution is required, since the control group plays the most important but, at the same time, the most sensitive and vulnerable role in the quantitation of functional neuroimaging.

We will encounter this problem in some of the functional neuroimaging studies in whiplash injury (see Sect. 3.2).

Current Research Data

3

3.1 Mild Traumatic Brain Injury

3.1.1 General Aspects

Traumatic brain injury is usually assessed with the Glasgow Coma Scale (GCS), CT, and EEG. However, also a considerable number of articles with functional neuroimaging can be retrieved on mild traumatic brain injury. Many of these document that in mild traumatic brain injury, SPET and PET imaging are superior to the morphologically oriented procedures – like CT or MRI – as SPET or PET can also image functionally altered cerebral regions. Often, these functional lesions are larger and more frequent than in the CT finding.

Jacobs et al. (1994) designed a study to answer the question of whether the aforementioned superiority of functional imaging was also relevant: They found that perfusion SPET has a high negative-predictive value for the clinical outcome. It was shown that with initially negative SPET findings, 97% of the patients did not have any clinical symptoms 3 months after a mild to moderate brain damage, while 95% with clinical symptoms 3 months after the accident had a positive initial SPET scan. These results are very important in terms of rehabilitation and for the evaluation of the ability of the patient to work.

In the study from Ichise et al. (1994), patients with chronic symptoms after traumatic brain injury were investigated utilizing perfusion SPET compared to neuropsychological testing. The presence of pathological SPET findings correlated with a set of neuropsychological tests. Especially, it was found that by the determination of the ratio of anterior to posterior brain perfusion, the degrees of the morphological deficits could be predicted. By contrast, the ventricle to cortex ratio correlated only weakly with the neuropsychological tests.

Compared to the work of Ichise and colleagues, a study on survivors of severe closed head injury from Goldenberg et al. (1992) revealed a far worse correlation of SPET with the neuropsychological tests. In this context, it should be noted that a normal SPET or PET does not necessarily have to exclude mild traumatic brain lesions, as a diffuse axonal damage to the brain cannot be imaged by these imaging modalities.

A. Otte, *Whiplash Injury*,
DOI 10.1007/978-3-642-28356-7_3, © Springer-Verlag Berlin Heidelberg 2012

In a combined ^{57}Co-/^{99m}Tc-HMPAO study, Audenaert et al. (2003) could show that ^{57}Co-SPET is able to outline the site and extent of brain damage in patients with mild traumatic brain injury, even in the absence of structural lesions and that it may confirm and localize findings from neuropsychological testing.

Goethals et al. (2004) studied the neural basis associated with performance on the Stroop Colored-Word test interference subtask in patients with diffuse brain injury using SPM and SPET. They could show that patients with diffuse brain injury were slower than healthy controls on the interference subtask of the Stroop test associated with activation effects in posterior (mainly parietal) brain areas in addition to activation of anterior (mainly anterior cingulate) brain regions.

3.1.2   Special Cases

The number of single cases and tragedies resulting from traumatic brain injuries is dramatic and could fill many books. We would, therefore, like to show some exemplary cases (data from Otte and Brändli 1998; Otte et al. 1998b).

3.1.2.1 Bicycle Accident

In this case, a 35-year-old man was referred to hospital after a bicycle accident where he had hit the right side of his head on the street. On the day of the accident, he complained of cervical pain, extraordinary right-hemispheric headache, dizziness, fluctuating vertigo, and visual symptoms (oscillopsia). Neuropsychological testing exhibited a marked reduction of attention and concentration for tonic and phasic alertness, for divided attention, and for the cognitive information processing speed. In addition, verbal and visuospatial memory was reduced. CT and MRI showed no pathological findings of the brain. The EEG revealed right-hemispheric general changes in the temporoparietal brain region. Using FDG-PET and SPM, a marked reduction of glucose utilization in the right frontal, parietal, and occipital region could be detected (Fig. 3.1).

One year after the accident, the patient had to give up his job due to persisting deficits in concentration, memory, and attention; he also had to stop his studies at university which he had started alongside his job. The headache, the visual symptoms, and the fluctuating vertigo attacks persisted.

Bicycle accidents can cause many kinds of injuries; the serious ones are mainly resulting from head impact (Thompson et al. 1989). Those patients with head injuries and negative brain CT or MRI, but persisting cerebral dysfunctions, are often judged to be malingerers despite the fact that quantitative functional neuroimaging, such as PET or SPET, demonstrates brain dysfunctions, as in the reported case.

3.1.2.2 Car Accident

A 47-year-old woman had a mild traumatic brain injury as a consequence of a rear-end car collision and subsequently developed a posttraumatic distress syndrome with changes of her personality and depression. She complained about mood changes, alterations in concentration and memory, sleep disturbances, occipital

Fig. 3.1 FDG-PET SPM image of a patient after bicycle accident showing a marked reduction of glucose utilization in the right frontal, parietal, and occipital region of the brain (This figure was published in Otte et al. (1998b), copyright Elsevier (1998). With kind reproduction permission from Elsevier Ltd.)

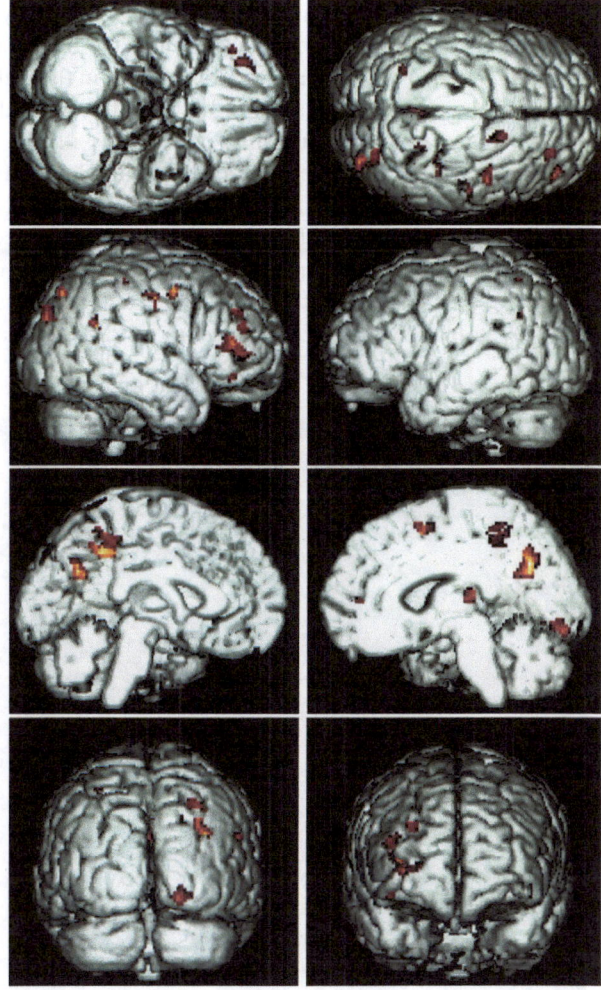

headache, vertigo, fluctuating visual disturbances, tendency towards aggressiveness, and fatigue.

The clinical investigation revealed a lateralization of Weber's test to the left ear from where it had bleeded after the accident. Furthermore, the patient had hyposmia at the right side for aromatic and trigeminal irritants. She also had a tender point at the third cervical spine and pain of the shoulders and neck. ^{99m}Tc-ECD (Neurolite) SPET 20 months after the accident showed hypoperfusion in the right posterior parietal occipital and in the right frontobasal regions (Fig. 3.2a).

In a follow-up investigation 44 months after the accident, an improvement of the patient's cervical, neck, and shoulder pain and a disappearance of the fluctuating visual disturbances and occipital headaches were observed. Tests for memory and concentration were normal. By contrast, her tendency towards aggressiveness did not change, and the hyposmia at the right side turned into anosmia. The follow-up ECD-SPET scan revealed a normal perfusion in the right posterior parietal occipital region, but a clear accentuation of the right frontobasal hypoperfusion (Fig. 3.2b).

In this case, brain perfusion is correlated with the patient's clinical symptoms. Hypoperfusion of the posterior parietal occipital region that is localized to the watershed zone between the territories of the larger cerebral arteries may be the substrate of the cognitive and visual disturbances in the reported patient, as the parietal and occipital regions have functions in the maintenance of attention and in complex sensory processing (Mesulam 1985). Frontal lesions are well known to cause changes in personality, as well as frontobasal lesions are related with hyposmia or

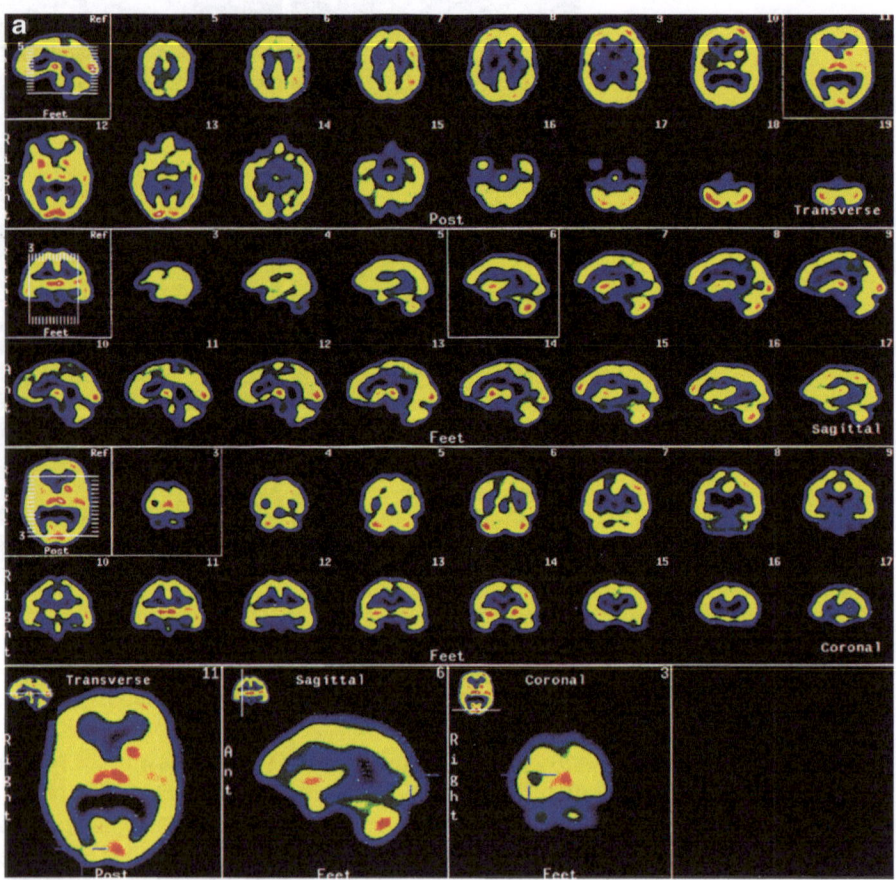

Fig. 3.2 Perfusion SPET (^{99m}Tc-ECD [Neurolite]) in a patient with car accident and mild traumatic brain injury: (**a**) 20 months after the accident showing hypoperfusion in the right posterior parietal occipital and right frontobasal region and (**b**) 44 months after the accident showing a normal perfusion in the right posterior parietal occipital region, but a clear accentuation of the right frontobasal hypoperfusion (These figures were published in Otte and Brändli (1998), copyright Elsevier (1998). With kind reproduction permission from Elsevier Ltd.)

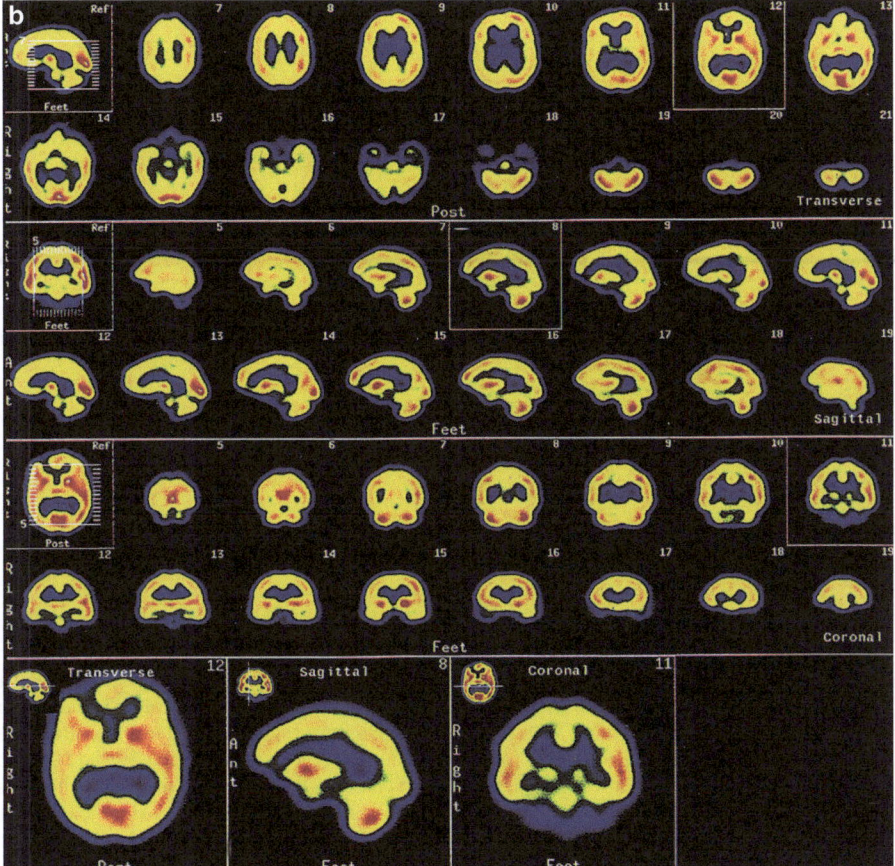

Fig. 3.2 (continued)

anosmia. In the reported case, the lesions in the frontobasal and posterior parietal occipital region at the right side can be explained by brain contusions as a consequence of a coup-contrecoup mechanism. Interestingly, the posterior parietal occipital lesion disappears, whereas the frontobasal defect accentuates. This emphasizes both the plasticity and the susceptibility of the brain to contusion mechanisms.

3.2 Whiplash Injury

In comparison to literature data on mild traumatic brain injury, the bibliography on whiplash injury and late whiplash injury is slightly smaller, albeit persistently increasing over the last few years. This may also result from the practice that sometimes studies of whiplash injury are entitled studies of mild traumatic brain injury. Still, PET or SPET data in whiplash brain are rare, however, and currently only available mainly from data of a small number of research groups.

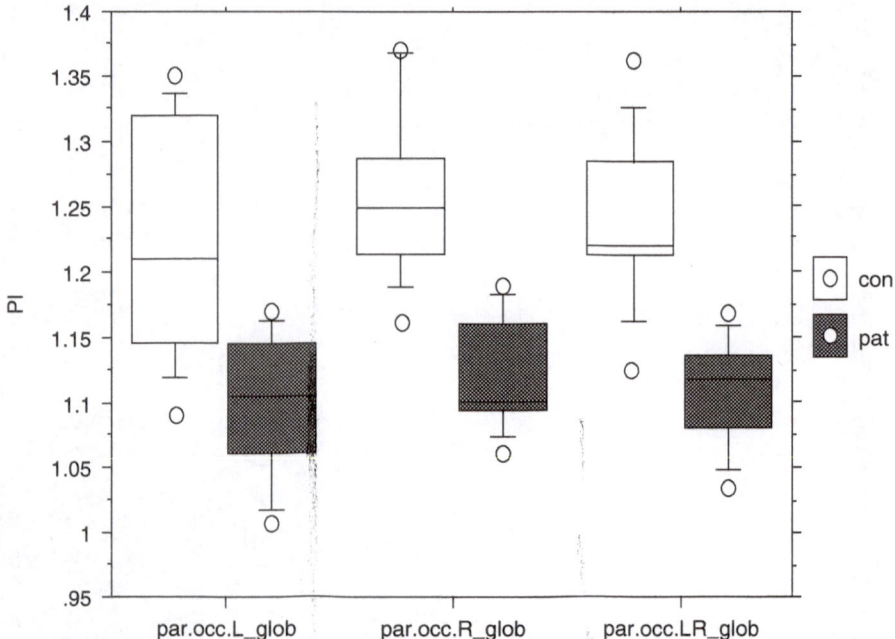

Fig. 3.3 Box plot of the perfusion indices in the posterior parietal occipital region related to the global perfusion at height of basal ganglia determined by perfusion SPET (^{99m}Tc-ECD) and region-of-interest technique. Ten patients with late whiplash syndrome are compared to 11 controls. par. occ.L_glob means the perfusion index for the posterior parietal occipital region related to global for the left side, par.occ.R_glob for the right side, and par.occ.LR_glob for the means of both sides: con=control group, pat=patient group. The investigation resulted in statistically significant differences between the patient and the control group (Mann–Whitney U test) (par.occ.L_glob con-pat: $P=0.0031$; par.occ.R_glob con-pat: $P=0.0002$; and par.occ.LR_glob: $P=0.0003$) (Originally from Otte et al. 1996a, adapted from Otte (2001) Das Halswirbelsäulen-Schleudertrauma: Neue Wege der funktionellen Bildgebung des Gehirns - Ein Ratgeber für Ärzte und Betroffene, Springer, Heidelberg)

Over the last years, Otte et al. (1995a, b, 1996a, b, 1997a, b, c, d, 1998a; Otte 1998, 1999, 2000a, d, 2001a, b, c) have performed several studies with SPET and PET using different tracers (^{99m}Tc-labeled HMPAO, ^{99m}Tc-labeled ECD, and ^{18}F-labeled FDG). In these studies, altogether over 500 patients with late whiplash syndrome were investigated at rest. With many of these patients, a – compared to a healthy control group – statistically significant relative reduction of the tracer in the posterior parietal occipital region, mostly affecting both sides, was seen (Fig. 3.3).

The aforementioned finding of hypoperfusion/hypometabolism in the posterior parietal occipital region could be reproduced by utilization of different SPET systems (dual-headed, triple-headed camera), different filter systems, different tracers (HMPAO, ECD, FDG), and different kinds of image interpretation such as visual analysis, semiquantitative ROI technique, and the observer-independent SPM procedure (Otte et al. 1995a, b, 1996a, b, 1997a, b, c, d, 1998a; Otte 1998, 1999, 2000a, d, 2001a, b, c).

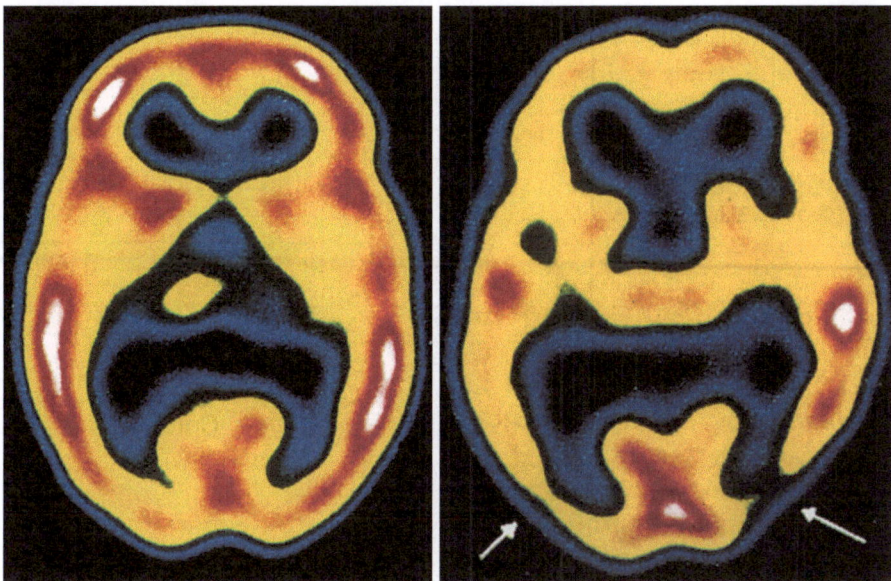

Fig. 3.4 Late whiplash syndrome, example 1: *Left*: Normal control and *right*: whiplash patient with persisting symptoms 2 years after accident. Representative transaxial slices at level of basal ganglia: perfusion SPET. A perfusion reduction can be seen on both sides of the posterior parietal occipital region, see *arrows* (This figure was published in Otte et al. (1997a), copyright Elsevier (1997). With kind reproduction permission from Elsevier Ltd.)

In addition, in individual cases, there was a tracer reduction in regions apart from the posterior parietal occipital region, e.g., in the frontal and/or temporal lobe. These changes were, however, not group-specifically significant, i.e., the whiplash patient group did not have the common characteristic of a perfusion reduction in the frontal or temporal region; however, an individual patient compared to a control group could have statistically significant perfusion reductions in these regions.

Some neuroimaging SPET examples of patients with late whiplash syndrome are presented in Figs. 3.4 and 3.5.

In a study from 1997 (Otte et al. 1997b), 6 whiplash patients as well as 12 normal controls were examined both by SPET (perfusion tracer ^{99m}Tc-ECD) and PET (glucose metabolism tracer ^{18}F-FDG). Standardized elliptical regions of interest were placed in various *Talairach*-standardized transaxial slices in different brain regions and normalized to the perfusion and glucose utilization in height of the basal ganglia (resulting in the perfusion index and glucose metabolic index). In both assessments, a statistically significant and matching decrease in perfusion/metabolism was found in the posterior parietal occipital region of both brain sides. This decrease was group specific; in individual cases, also other regions of significantly decreased perfusion/metabolism were observed, such as in the frontal, parietal, and temporal lobe or in the brain stem. However, there were no statistically significant group differences in these additional brain regions (Figs. 3.6 and 3.7).

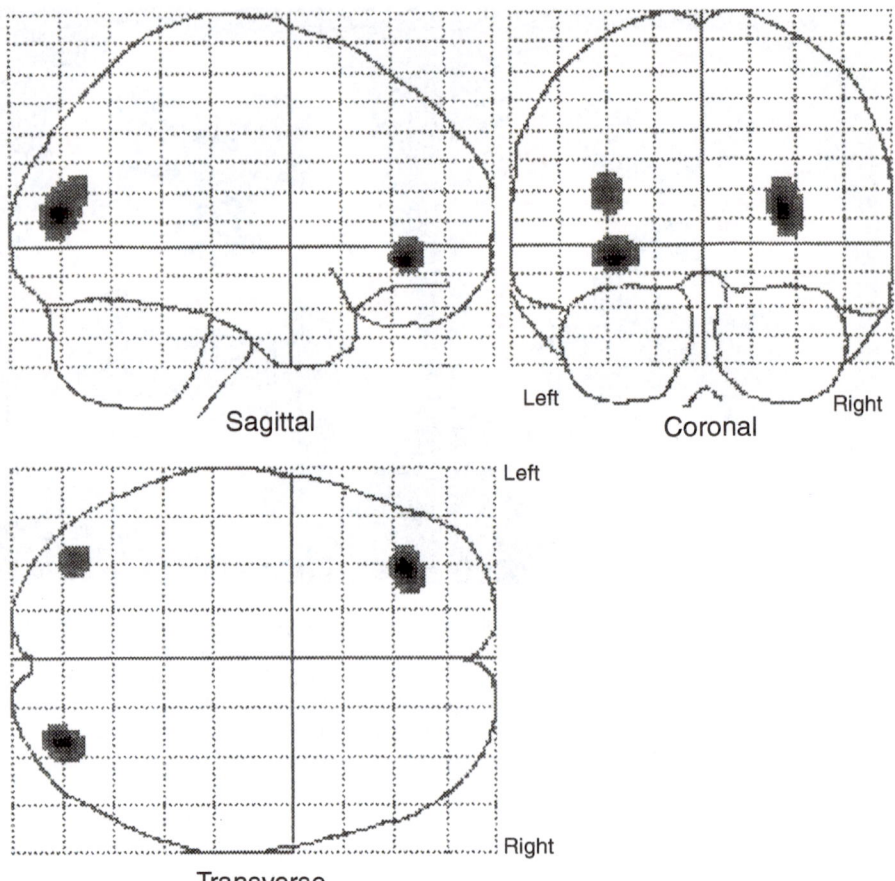

Sagittal

Left   Right

Coronal

Left

Transverse

Right

Fig. 3.5 Late whiplash syndrome, example 2: Statistical parametric map projections; brain areas with significantly decreased relative perfusion (level of significance: $p < 0.01$) of 15 whiplash patients compared to 15 healthy controls are shown; from these 15 whiplash patients, all could remember that they had looked to the right during the impact; 10 patients reported that they had hit their heads at the steering wheel. Statistically significant differences are displayed on sagittal, coronal, and transaxial projections of the brain: ^{99m}Tc-ECD-SPET. Note the hypoperfusion in the posterior parietal occipital region at both sides and in the frontal region on the left side; the hypoperfusion frontal left – posterior parietal occipital right – may be explained by a traumatic coup-contrecoup mechanism, whereas the additional hypoperfusion in the posterior parietal occipital region on the left side can only be explained by the additional whiplash injury (Originally from Otte et al. 1998a, adapted from Otte et al. (eds) (2004) Nuclear Medicine in Psychiatry, Springer, Heidelberg)

It is hypothesized that the hypometabolism in the posterior parietal occipital region is caused by activation of nociceptive afferents from the upper cervical spine. This hypothesis is based on a study by Moskowitz and Buzzi (1991) from which it is known that irritation of nociceptive afferents of the projections of the trigeminal nerve has different effects on local vasoactive peptides and the cranial blood vessel

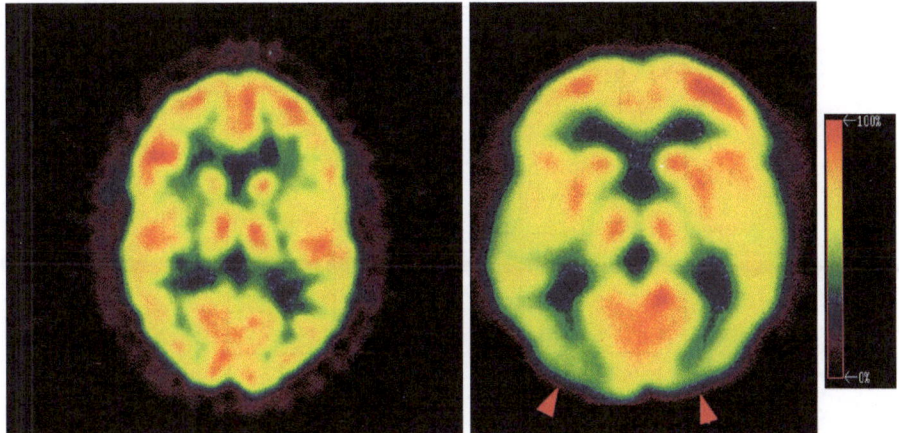

Fig. 3.6 FDG-PET; representative transaxial slice in height of basal ganglia, *left*: normal control subject, *right*: whiplash patient; *arrows* indicate hypometabolism in the posterior parietal occipital region (Data from Otte et al. 1997b, adapted from Otte et al. (eds) (2004) Nuclear Medicine in Psychiatry, Springer, Heidelberg)

system. The fact that the posterior brain perfusion area, in particular the area of the terminal vascular bed between the A. cerebri media and the A. cerebri posterior (which is primarily the posterior parietal occipital region) is mainly affected, can be explained by the knowledge that this area is attributed one of the most vulnerable regions of the brain (Graham and Brierly 1984; Otte 2000d).

To test the hypothesis of nociceptive afferences versus contusion mechanism, Otte et al. (1998) reevaluated their large group of whiplash patients scanned with ^{99m}Tc-ECD SPET and found 15 patients who themselves drived their cars and who all could remember that they looked to the right side when the rear-end car collision happened. Ten of the 15 patients reported that they had hit their heads on the steering wheel, and the other five could not remember. Otte et al. checked these 15 patients against 15 age- and sex-matched healthy volunteers using SPM96.

The whiplash patients revealed a significant hypoperfusion in the posterior parietal occipital region of both hemispheres and in the left frontal region (Fig. 3.5).

As the patients looked to the right side during the accident, a contusion mechanism could be discussed for the left frontal and the right posterior parietal occipital region, regardless if this was produced directly by hitting the head to the steering wheel or by the acceleration forces producing indirect head impact. If whiplash injury only was a form of mild head injury with a contusion mechanism, the additional left posterior parietal occipital hypoperfusion in the above patients could not be explained. Therefore, the authors conclude that posterior parietal occipital hypoperfusion in whiplash patients may still be hypothesized to be elicited from lesions of neuroceptive afferents from the upper cervical spine. Of course, this does not exclude, so the authors, that brain contusions must carefully be evaluated, as additional contusion is well known to have an effect on clinical outcome after injury.

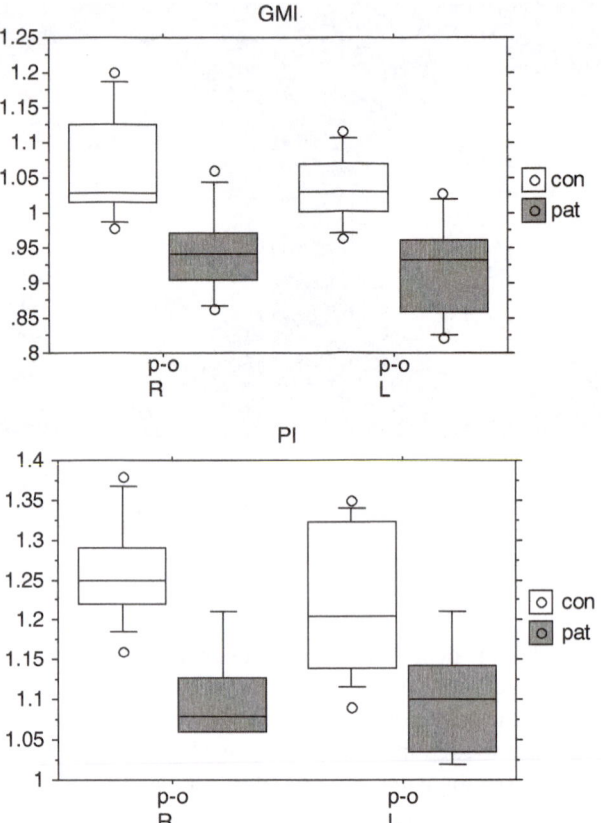

Fig. 3.7 *Above*: box plot of the glucose metabolic indices (GMI) determined by ^{18}F-FDG-PET and region-of-interest technique in the posterior parietal occipital region related to the global glucose metabolism at height of the basal ganglia. *Below*: box plot of the perfusion indices (PI) determined by ^{99m}Tc-ECD. Six whiplash patients were compared with 12 controls in both assessments. p-o L means posterior parietal occipital region left, and p-o R, posterior parietal occipital region right: con=control group, pat=patient group. The investigation resulted in statistically significant differences between the patient and the control group both in the GMI and the PI values (Mann–Whitney *U* test) (*GMI*: p-o R con-pat: *P*=0.0092, p-o L con-pat: *P*=0.0067; *PI*: p-o R con-pat: *P*=0.0039, p-o L con-pat: *P*=0.0273) (Data from Otte et al. 1997b, adapted from Otte et al. (eds) (2004) Nuclear Medicine in Psychiatry, Springer, Heidelberg)

In addition, in head injury, the typical contusion regions of postmortem brains have been investigated already by Courville, in 1937 (Courville 1937). These are shown in Fig. 3.8, and it can be seen that the posterior parietal occipital region is not a contusion localization in traumatic brain injury.

In a study with FDG-PET, HMPAO-SPET, and MRI, Bicik et al. (1998) examined a small sample size of 13 patients with "typical whiplash syndrome." They compared the PET and SPET data, however not the MRI data, with 16 controls. The controls comprised four healthy students and twelve melanoma patients.

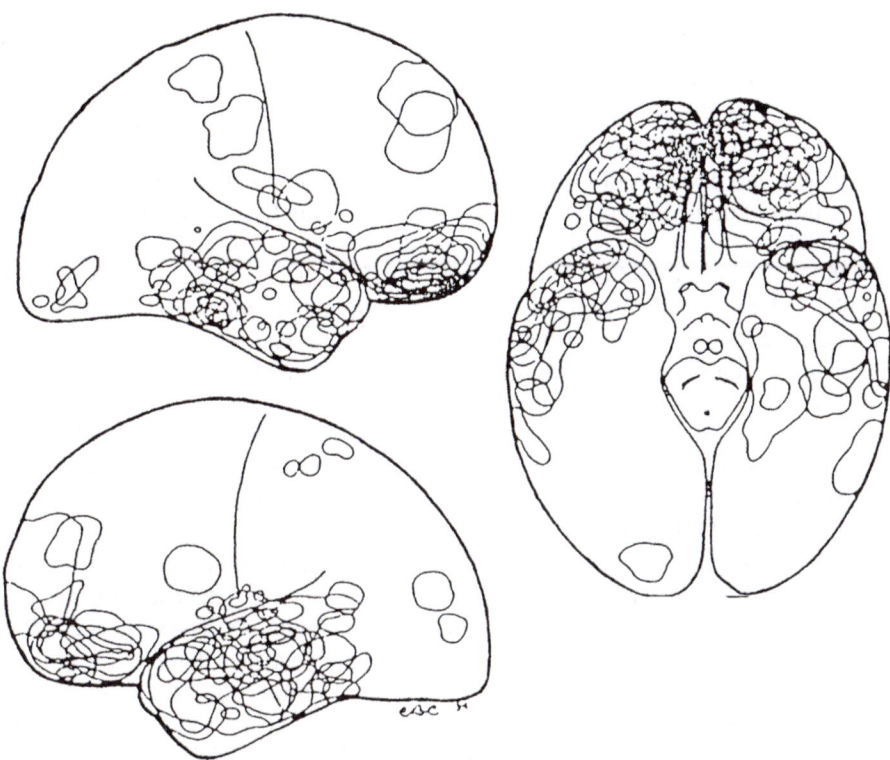

Fig. 3.8 Pathological-anatomical distribution of the localizations involved in brain contusion subsequent to closed head injury (adapted from Courville 1937). The frontal and temporal regions are most frequently affected. The posterior parietal occipital region, which can be altered after whiplash injury, is not affected. For this, a different mechanism must be postulated (Adapted from Otte (2001) Das Halswirbelsäulen-Schleudertrauma: Neue Wege der funktionellen Bildgebung des Gehirns - Ein Ratgeber für Ärzte und Betroffene, Springer, Heidelberg)

The group found by SPM a significantly decreased metabolism in the frontopolar, temporolateral region, as well as in the putamen. The frontopolar changes correlated significantly with the Beck Depression Inventory scale. In the posterior parietal occipital region, a decreased perfusion and glucose utilization was found, but this hypometabolism correlated with a cortical thinning in the MRI. Based on their small sample size, the group concluded that the FDG-PET or HMPAO-SPET was not recommendable as diagnostic routine investigation for whiplash patients.

This study was discussed in one of the later issues of the journal where it was published with a reply by one of the authors representatively for the working group (Otte 1999; Buck 1999). In this scientific discussion, it was pointed out that the control group consisted mainly of melanoma patients, a group of patients, thus, who exhibit neuropsychological changes high-probably alone due to emotion-related cognitive changes based on the awareness of their cancer illness. A neuropsychological testing to exclude any bias with this was, unfortunately, not performed for this so-called "control" group. Moreover, in a study from Tashiro et al. (2000), SPM and FDG PET impressively revealed statistically significant brain alterations (mainly in the frontal and parietal regions) in oncological patients (see also Sect. 2.5).

Furthermore, the study by Bicik et al. did not perform an MRI of the brains of the control group. Exactly, this is, however, the main weak point of the study: It would have been of utmost interest to compare the cortical thickness to the brain perfusion also in the control group. This would have helped to find out if the cortical thickness in the posterior parietal occipital region, which in the patient group did correlate with the decreased perfusion, was equal or not equal between controls and patients. Hence, the key question of whether the posterior parietal occipital region is functionally or morphologically "thinned" in whiplash patients remains unanswered in this study.

The study group of the article from Radanov et al. (1999) consists of nearly the same members as the one by Bicik and coworkers. The difference to the publication of Bicik et al. lies in the addition of neuropsychological testing to the functional neuroimaging PET and SPET. Radanov et al. found that whiplash patients have positive findings in neuropsychological tests for cognitive functions, but no significant correlation between the regional brain perfusion or the glucose utilization and the scores in the tests of divided attention or working memory. The authors conclude that in late whiplash syndrome, there is no correlation between diagnosable morphological or functional brain deficits and cognitive functions; they, therefore, surmise that the emotional and cognitive symptoms are triggered but not caused by the whiplash injury. Most of this, however, contradicts to the work by Ichise et al. (1994).

An editorial by Alexander (1998) states that a pure whiplash injury can cause a traumatic brain injury and that functional brain deficits can be measured subsequent to whiplash injury; however, Alexander is not in favor of the application of SPET, even if correlated to neuropsychological tests, for the verification of the cause of the brain lesion. Poeck (1999) states that the new functional imaging data are not recommendable for the diagnosis of the late whiplash syndrome. Both, Alexander and Poeck, base their argumentation on the study from Bicik et al., in which case, as we think, a critical approach to the interpretation of their comments should be taken (Otte 2000d).

By contrast, in a recent study from Lorberboym et al. (2002), 20 patients with late whiplash syndrome were investigated with HMPAO-SPET and tests of perception and cognition including the P300 (an electrophysiological marker of cognitive ability), the digit span test, the word list generation test, two bedside memory tests, the Hamilton Depression Rating Scale, the Hamilton Anxiety Scale, and the Rivermead Postconcussion Symptoms questionnaire. A control group of nine volunteers without whiplash or head trauma was also tested. The authors found the following interesting results, which are also important for the validity of the aforementioned studies by Otte et al.:

- While no structural brain damage was seen in any patient on MRI, 13 of the 20 patients had brain perfusion abnormalities in one or more regions: Eight of these 13 patients had decreased perfusion in the temporal lobes, 3 patients had occipital perfusion abnormalities, 2 patients showed frontal lobe abnormalities, and 2 patients had asymmetric perfusion in the basal ganglia.

- Eight of 15 patients had abnormal P300 studies, and 7 of these 8 patients with abnormal P300 results had also an abnormal SPET study. From the 7 of 15 patients with normal P300 results, 6 had a normal SPET.
- Although there was no significant correlation between the SPET findings or the P300 results and the scores of attention and working memory, there was a close agreement between the SPET and P300 findings.

Data from larger patient collectives on the diagnostics of the late whiplash syndrome by using functional MRI or magnetic resonance spectroscopy to the best of our knowledge still do not exist, although they would certainly be desirable. However, we know of one encouraging pilot study in five symptomatic patients with late

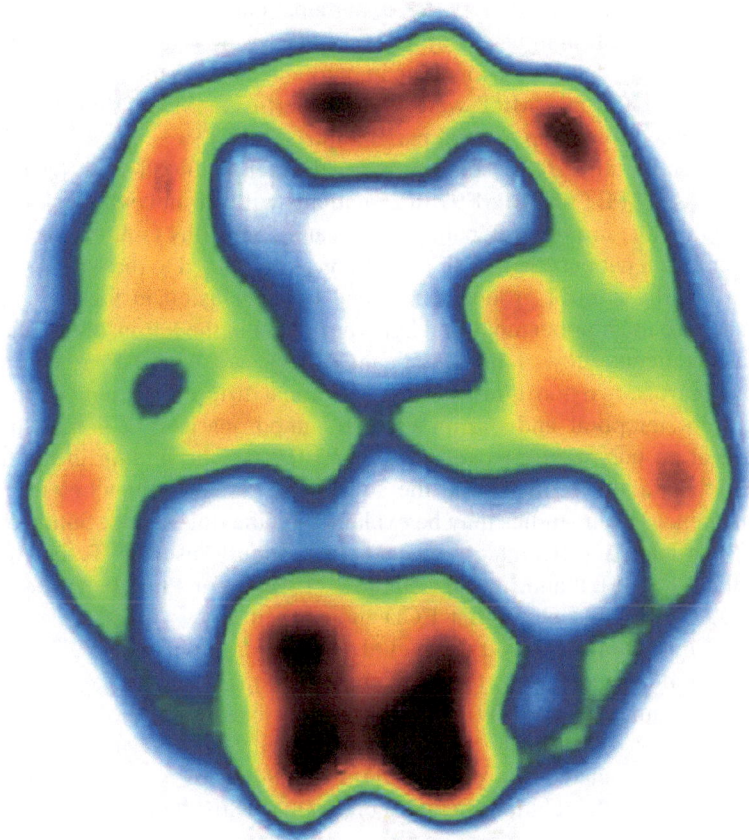

Fig. 3.9 Posterior type of hypoperfusion in a patient after whiplash injury (This figure was published in Lass and Lyczak (2004), with kind permission from the *Hellenic Journal of Nuclear Medicine*, Thessaloniki)

whiplash syndrome, five asymptomatic patients after whiplash trauma, and a control group of seven volunteers without the history of trauma; in this study, tests for visual motion perception and functional MRI measurements during visual motion stimulation were performed (Freitag et al. 2001). Symptomatic patients presented a significant reduction in their ability to perceive coherent visual motion compared to controls, whereas the asymptomatic patients did not show this effect; functional MRI activation was similar during random dot motion in all three groups, but was significantly decreased during coherent dot motion in the symptomatic patients compared with the other two groups. Reduced psychophysical motion performance and reduced functional MRI responses in symptomatic patients with late whiplash syndrome suggest a functional impairment in cortical areas sensitive to coherent motion. These findings in visual motion perception are in accordance with the SPET and PET findings in the posterior parietal occipital region and present a first and important proof of evidence of these cerebral findings by another imaging method.

In 2004, Lass and Lyczak reported about a patient aged 46 years who had a car accident with whiplash injury, without a loss of consciousness. This patient, so the authors, gradually developed cognitive impairment and was unable to come back to work. Whereas CT and MRT were normal, perfusion SPET showed significant hypoperfusion of the temporal and parietal lobes (Fig. 3.9).

Sundström et al. (2006) studied regional cerebral blood flow (rCBF) using ^{99m}Tc-HMPAO SPET and SPM'99 in 27 patients with chronic whiplash syndrome, 18 nontraumatic chronic neck pain patients, and 15 healthy controls. The nontraumatic neck pain patients had rCBF alterations as compared to the whiplash patients and the healthy control group, comprising hypoperfusion in the right temporal region near to the hippocampus and hyperperfusion in the left insula. Although the whiplash patients showed no significant differences in rCBF as compared to healthy controls, two nonsignificant small regional differences could be found, one in the right temporal and one in the left temporoparietal region, which were detected at an uncorrected voxel level of $P=0.001$. The finding in the left temporoparietal region (representing the somatosensory area) matches our studies. The difference to our studies may be explained by the tracer used: Sundström et al. used ^{99m}Tc-HMPAO (Ceretec), whereas we mainly used ^{99m}Tc-labeled ECD (Neurolite) for SPET and, in later studies, ^{18}F-FDG for PET. In a study already from 1997, we could show that ECD more often shows functional changes in whiplash injury than HMPAO (Otte et al. 1997a), an observation which has been seen also in other indications for functional neuroimaging.

Recently, Linnman et al. (2009) studied two objectives in whiplash injury:

1. To compare resting state rCBF by ^{15}O-labeled H_2O PET in 21 patients with whiplash-associated disorders (WAD) with 18 healthy, pain-free controls
2. To investigate the relations between brain areas with altered rCBF to pain experience, somatic symptoms, posttraumatic stress symptoms, and personality traits in the patient group

The group found elevated rCBF bilaterally in the posterior parahippocampal and the posterior cingulate gyri, in the right thalamus and the right medial prefrontal gyrus compared to healthy controls. Furthermore, they found lowered rCBF in the temporo-occipital regions compared to healthy controls.

These alterations in rCBF in the patients were correlated with neck disability ratings.

The authors concluded that there was an involvement of the posterior cingulate, parahippocampal, and medial prefrontal gyri in patients with WAD and speculated that changes in the resting state were linked to an increased self-relevant evaluation of pain and stress. Hyperperfusion in these areas was not systematically investigated in the past studies from Otte et al. (1995a, b, 1996a, b, 1997a, b, c, d, e, 1998a, b, c, d) and others. At that time only hypoperfusion was looked at due to the cognitive deficits reported in late whiplash syndrome.

Clas Linnman's reported relatively lower rCBF in the temporo-occipital areas are, however, consistent with the findings reported by Otte et al. (1995a, b, 1996a, b, 1997a, b, c, d, e, 1998a, b, c, d). Linnman and his coworkers state that these findings have also been observed in experimental models of pain. This is in accordance with the hypothesis from Otte et al. (1995a, b, 1996a, b, 1997a, b, c, d, e, 1998a, b, c, d) that neuroceptive afferents may be responsible for vasopeptide-induced vasoconstriction in the posterior parietal occipital regions (which is in the posterior watershed zone of the brain), as described by Moskowitz and Buzzi 1991 and Otte 2012.

Apart from rCBF, Linnman et al. (2010, 2012) have studied the substance P neurokinin-1 (NK1) receptor availability in patients with grade II whiplash-associated disorder using ^{11}C-GR205171 PET.

The group found reduced NK1 receptor availability in the ventromedial prefrontal, the insular and cingulate cortex, the hippocampus, the amygdala, and the periaqueductal gray area (Linnman et al. 2010).

In addition, Linnman et al. (2012) recently revisited their aforementioned (2010) data to investigate the brain NK1 receptor availability in the posterior parietal occipital region of whiplash patients and found a significantly reduced NK1 receptor availability in the left middle occipital gyrus, the right middle temporal gyrus, the left superior temporal gyrus, and the right superior temporal gyrus (Fig. 3.10).

These new data add further evidence to the original findings by Otte et al. in the posterior parietal occipital region of the brain after whiplash injury.

A further interesting study from Linnman and colleagues has been published (Linnman et al. 2011), which aims at investigating neck inflammation in patients with whiplash-associated disorders. In this PET study, the ^{11}C-labeled inflammation marker S-(+)-(d)-D-deprenyl is used. It could be shown that whiplash patients had a significantly increased ^{11}C-D deprenyl uptake in the area surrounding the spinous process of the second cervical vertebra (Fig. 3.11), suggesting persistent musculoskeletal inflammation in this region.

Last but not least, a detailed German compendium on whiplash injury can be found in Graf et al. (2009), comprising a series of general aspects on anatomy, physiology, neurobiology, and psychology; on biomechanics; and on diagnostic and

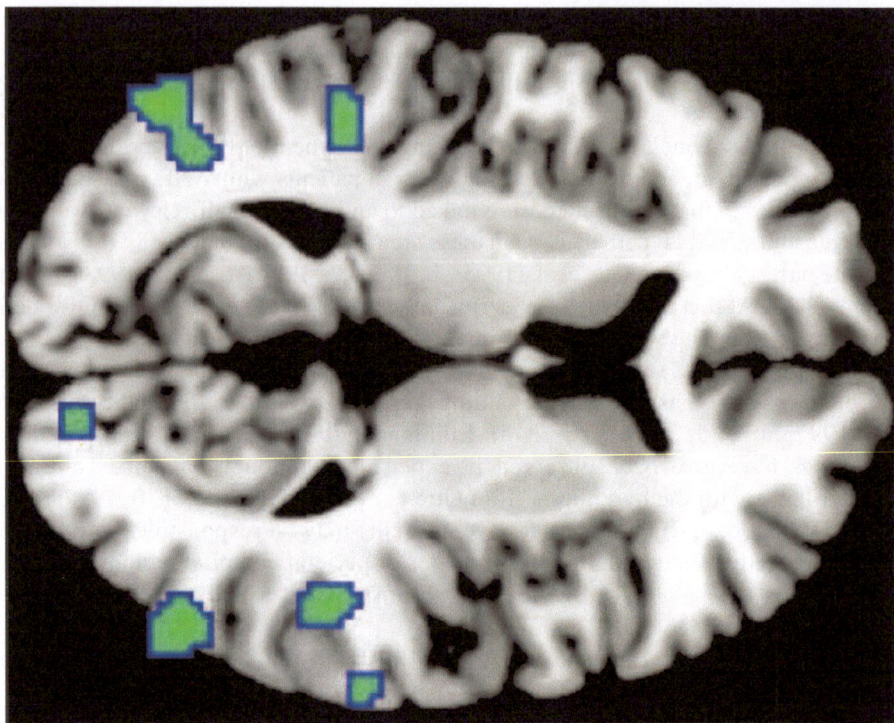

Fig. 3.10 Neurokinin-1 receptor availability imaged with ^{11}C-GR205171 PET in 18 patients with grade II whiplash-associated disorder compared to 18 healthy controls, region-of-interest analysis (statistical parametric mapping, SPM2) restricted to the temporal, occipital, and parietal lobe. The results are uncorrected for multiple comparisons and displayed on an MRI template at $P<0.001$ (This figure is published in Linnman et al. (2012). With kind permission from Dr. Clas Linnman, P.A.I.N. Group, McLean Hospital, Harvard Medical School, U.S.A., and the *European Journal of Pain*, Elsevier Ltd. and John Wiley & Sons Ltd. (after the journal has transferred))

therapeutic approaches. In addition, a special focus of this book is on legal aspects and details in the German setting.

3.3   Differential Diagnostic List

The effect of posterior parietal occipital hypoperfusion is impaired spatial ability and blurred vision; it may also cause difficulty in forming thoughts and difficulties not in attending but in disengaging attention once the subject has focussed on an object of attention (Posner and Dehaene 1994).

Lesions in the posterior parietal occipital region can also be found in other diseases, such as the systemic lupus erythematosus (Fig. 3.12; Otte et al. 1997e, 1998d; Weiner et al. 2000; Weiner and Otte 2004), multi-infarct dementia, vascular encephalopathy, sleep apnea syndrome (Miller et al. 1990), cerebral hypoxia (Miller et al. 1990), migraine with aura (Friberg 1991), or Alzheimer's disease

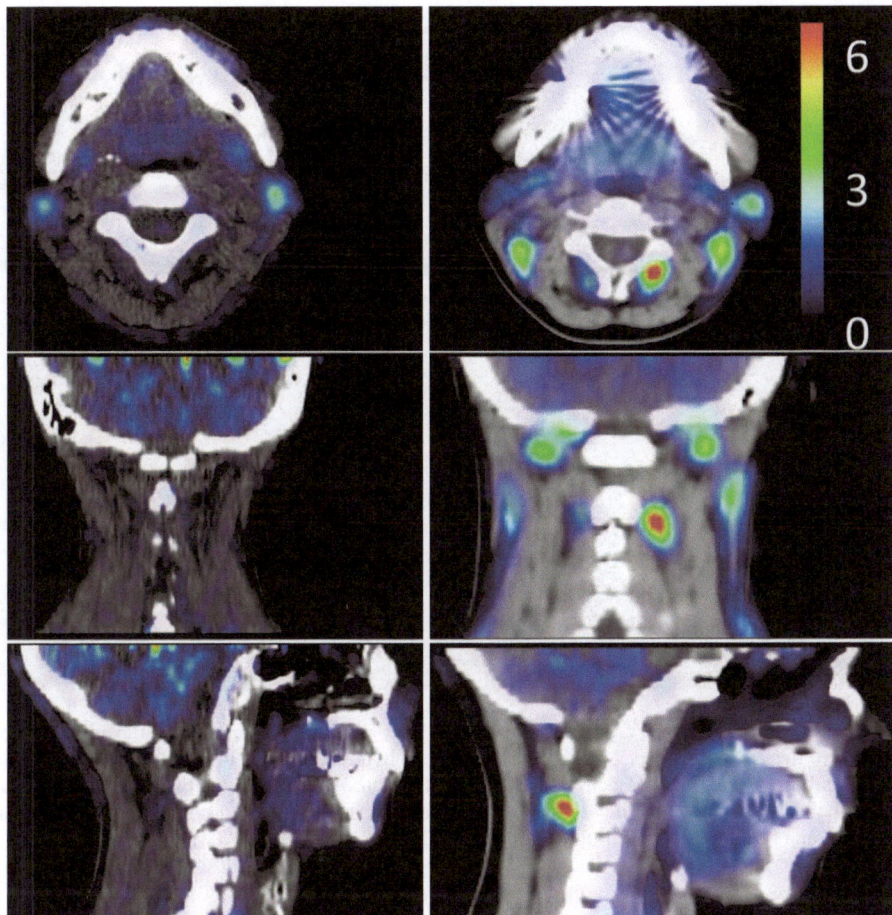

Fig. 3.11 ^{11}C-D deprenyl uptake in a representative healthy control (*left*) and in a patient with whiplash-associated disorders. ^{11}C-D deprenyl PET images are fusioned with the subject's individual CT scans. ^{11}C-D deprenyl uptake is expressed as standardized uptake value (SUV, see color bar in the figure). A high ^{11}C-D deprenyl uptake can be seen in the patient's adipose tissue preponderantly on the right side of the spinous process of the second cervical vertebra (This figure was published in Linnman et al. (2011). With kind permission from Dr. Clas Linnman, P.A.I.N. Group, McLean Hospital, Harvard Medical School, U.S.A.; open-access license from *PlosOne*, www.plosone.org)

(Waldemar et al. 1994). Due to this long differential diagnostic list, the findings in the late whiplash syndrome are disputed. By a purposeful clinical, serological and/or neurological assessment, the aforementioned other diseases can easily be teased out, however.

It is sometimes stated that whiplash patients – having similar symptoms, especially in cognitive functions, as fibromyalgia patients – have their symptoms based on an underlying fibromyalgia which was already present prior to the whiplash injury. However, a study by Otte et al. (1998c) in this patient group revealed by SPM

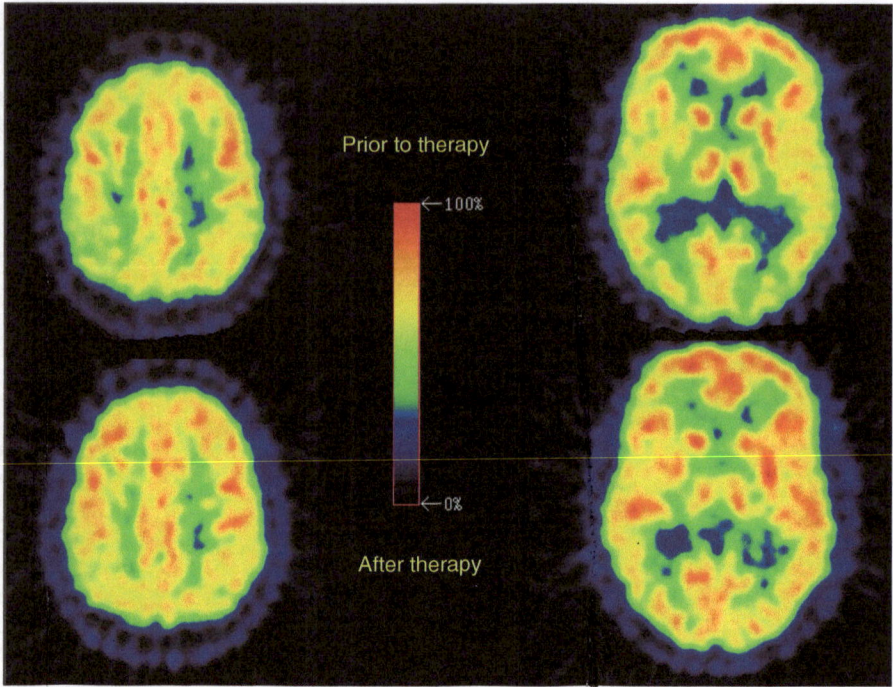

Fig. 3.12 Systemic lupus erythematosus. FDG-PET prior to (*upper row*) and after immunosuppressive therapy (*lower row*). Prior to the treatment, hypometabolism in the right parietal region and both posterior parietal occipital regions can be seen. After therapy, all regions have normal metabolism. Right image side = left brain side and vice versa (This figure has been published in Otte et al. (1998d), by SAGE Publications Ltd., all rights reserved, ©SAGE)

and SPET a statistically significant hypoperfusion in the frontal lobe at both sides, in the right temporal lobe, and in the head of the right caudate nucleus (Fig. 3.13). The results of this study are in keeping with other studies (e.g., Johansson et al. 1995; Costa et al. 1995; Costa and Greco 2004). Lesions in the posterior parietal occipital region were not found in fibromyalgia.

Also, the primary depression is stated as a cause for the late whiplash syndrome (e.g., Alexander 1998). SPET and PET alterations in the primary depression are, however, located primarily in the frontal lobe and not in the posterior parietal occipital region (e.g., Liotti and Mayberg 2001).

3.4   Whiplash Trauma and the Risk of Alzheimer's Disease

Interestingly, the cerebral hypometabolism in the posterior parietal occipital region, which we can observe in late whiplash syndrome, can also be found in Alzheimer's disease (Fig. 3.14).

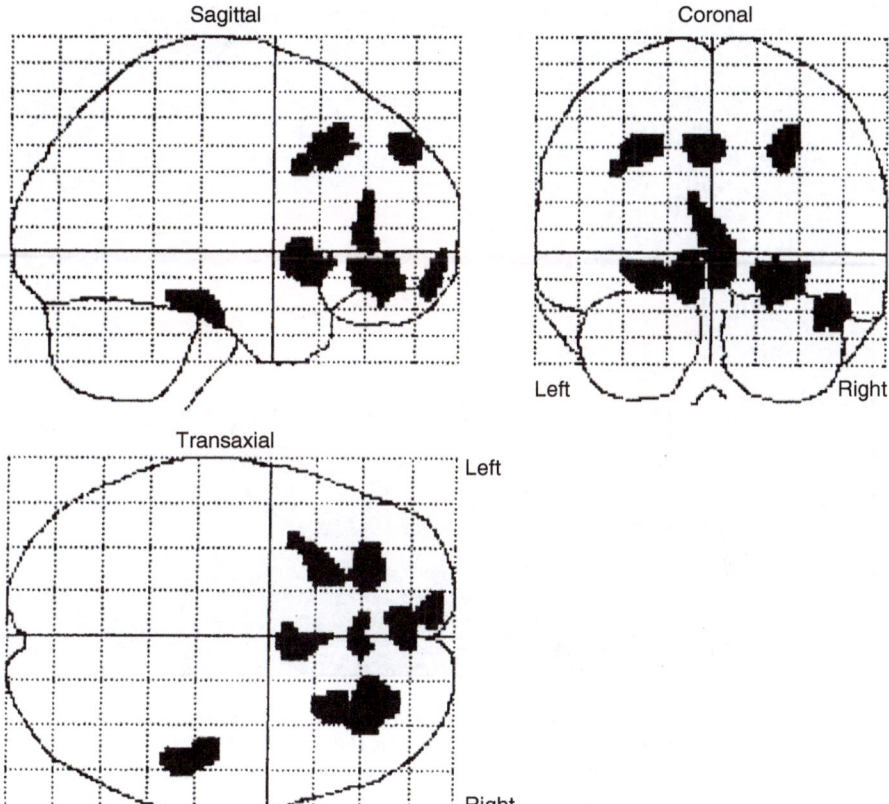

Fig. 3.13 Statistical parametric map projections showing significantly decreased brain perfusion (*P*-level < 0.01) in 18 patients with fibromyalgia syndrome versus 15 healthy volunteers. Differences are displayed on sagittal, coronal, and transaxial projections: ^{99m}Tc-ECD-SPET (This figure was published in Otte et al. (1998c), copyright Elsevier (1998). With kind reproduction permission from Elsevier Ltd.)

In the literature, there is some evidence of a link between head injury and the subsequent onset of Alzheimer's disease (Otte 1998).

Deposits of amyloid β-proteins cannot only be found in cases of dementia pugillistica (the boxers' disease), but are reported in some cases of patients dying after a single episode of severe head injury (Graham et al. 1996). Tang et al. (1996) found a tenfold increase in the risk of Alzheimer's disease associated with apolipoprotein E ε4 in combination with a history of traumatic head injury, compared to a twofold increase in risk with apolipoprotein E ε4 alone, whereas head injury in the absence of an apolipoprotein E ε4 allele did not increase the risk.

As shown, due to head restraints of today's cars, whiplash injury can also produce a head impact which may lead to direct brain damage and even pure whiplash trauma in rhesus monkeys without head restraints could be shown to generate direct

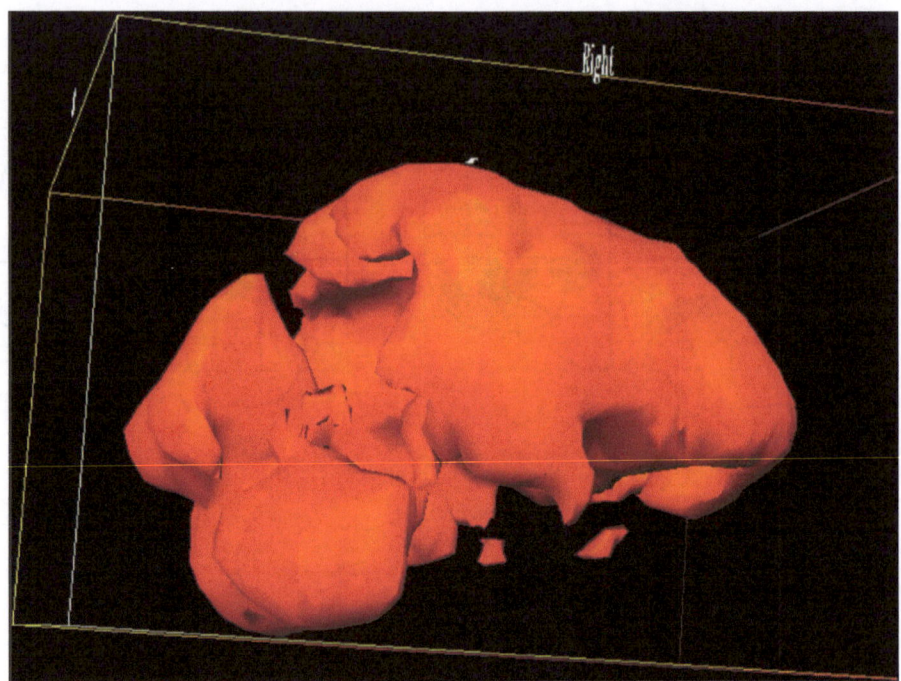

Fig. 3.14 Bilateral parietal/temporal hypoperfusion in Alzheimer's disease and perfusion SPET scan shown as 3D grid (Adapted from Otte (2001) Das Halswirbelsäulen-Schleudertrauma: Neue Wege der funktionellen Bildgebung des Gehirns - Ein Ratgeber für Ärzte und Betroffene, Springer, Heidelberg)

brain injury due to acceleration and deceleration forces (Ommaya et al. 1968). If severe head injury may trigger Alzheimer-disease-like pathology, an association or interaction with known genetic risk factors for Alzheimer's disease could be speculated in whiplash trauma (Otte 2004). However, this speculation needs to be confirmed by long-term multi-center studies and to date is not very likely. Certainly, a severe head injury is also not comparable with a whiplash injury.

Some authors do not support the hypothesis on exerting dementia of the Alzheimer's type by whiplash injury, e.g., Mehta et al. (1999) and Harwood et al. (1999). Mehta et al. (1999) performed a larger prospective study of a Rotterdam-based cohort of 6,645 patients finding no increased risk of dementia for patients with a history of head trauma. In addition, the apolipoprotein E ε4 allele did not modify this relationship.

The fascinating new world of DNA sequencing, which is available for the routine application setting since only few years, may provide further data on this interesting research field, which has also indeed become increasingly relevant today given the demographic development and the incidence of dementias.

Conclusion

4

Diagnostics of the late whiplash syndrome is a medically and legally challenging endeavor. So far, functional neuroimaging was neglected in contrast to morphological imaging tools, the latter being inconspicuous in most cases, the first showing significant deficits in the posterior parietal occipital region. Despite the findings in functional neuroimaging, the late whiplash syndrome remains a medical, political, ethical, and critical issue of actual concern.

Future animal research utilizing high-standard functional imaging devices and quality image analysis instruments may help to prove the causality of cerebral lesions in whiplash injury. In addition, new functional imaging modalities like functional MRI, magnetic resonance spectroscopy, MR/PET, or SQUID MEG should be introduced to preclinical and clinical research in the field.

Many whiplash patients had to give up their social lives, partnerships, and jobs. Not always are insurance claims the number one issue of their complaints. Frequently, their problems are subject to litigation or pushed – only little better – onto the psychological level.

It should be the primary aim of researchers and clinicians to find ways out of this dilemma.

A. Otte, *Whiplash Injury*,
DOI 10.1007/978-3-642-28356-7_4, © Springer-Verlag Berlin Heidelberg 2012

Clinical Aspects

5

Any physician involved, either directly or indirectly, in the problematic of whiplash patients should be aware of the preponderantly cerebral component of the late whiplash syndrome, leading to a puzzling diagnostic situation at the edge of a controversial medicolegal discussion. One way out of this situation is highly recommendable the thorough knowledge of recent research data on functional neuroimaging and its role in this indication. This may also help to understand how to best treat this patient population, which is still a challenge today. One approach, following the *Moskowitz* hypothesis, may be to eliminate the pain component of nociceptive afferents for the upper cervical spine, which – triggered by vasopeptides – may cause vasoconstriction in the posterior watershed zone, i.e., the posterior parietal occipital region.

Another approach may be to eliminate persistent peripheral tissue inflammation in the regions around the spinous process of the second cervical vertebra, as seen by Linnman et al. (2011) in a ^{11}C-D-deprenyl PET study (see Sect. 3.2).

This applies to any physician in the field, from the radiologist over the psychiatrist to the general practitioner. Also, different research groups, including experimental animal researchers, are highly encouraged to enrich this knowledge.

A. Otte, *Whiplash Injury*,
DOI 10.1007/978-3-642-28356-7_5, © Springer-Verlag Berlin Heidelberg 2012

References

Alexander MP (1998) In the pursuit of proof of brain damage after whiplash injury. Neurology 51:336–340

Audenaert K, Jansen HML, Otte A, Vervaet M, Crombez R, De Ridder L, Van Heeringen K, Dierckx RA, Korf J (2003) Imaging of mild traumatic brain injury using ^{57}Co and ^{99m}Tc HMPAO SPECT compared to conventional diagnostic procedures. Med Sci Monit 9:MT112–MT117

Barré JA (1926) Sur un syndrome sympathique cervical postérieur et sa cause fréquente. Lárthrite cervicale. Rev Neurol (Paris) 33:1246–1248

Bicik I, Radanov BP, Schäfer N, Dvorak J, Blum B, Weber B, Burger C, von Schulthess GK, Buck A (1998) PET with ^{18}fluorodeoxyglucose and hexamethylpropylene amine SPECT in late whiplash syndrome. Neurology 51:345–350

Buck A (1999) PET with ^{18}fluorodexyglucose and hexamethylpropylene amine oxime SPECT in late whiplash syndrome. Neurology 52:1108

Caplan EM (1995) Trains, brains, and sprains: railway spine and the origins of psychoneuroses. Bull Hist Med 69:387–419

Costa DC, Greco A (2004) Chronic fatigue syndrome/myalgic encephalomyelitis. In: Otte A, Audenaert K, Peremans K, Van Heering C, Dierckx RA (eds) Nuclear medicine in psychiatry. Springer, Berlin, Heidelberg, New York, Hong Kong, London, Milan, Paris, Tokyo, pp 289–300

Costa DC, Tannock C, Brostoff J (1995) Brainstem perfusion is impaired in chronic fatigue syndrome. QJM 88:767–773

Courville CB (1937) Pathology of the central nervous system. Mountain View, California Pacific

Croft AC (1998) Low speed rear impact collision (LOSRIC). In: Mürner J, Ettlin TM (Hrsg.) HWS-Distorsion (Schleudertrauma) und leichte traumatische Hirnverletzung. Medico-legal Congress, 25.-26.06.1998; Kongress-Band: 1–98

Elis A (2010) Mein Traum ist länger als die Nacht: Wie Bertha Benz ihren Mann zu Weltruhm fuhr. Hoffmann und Campe Verlag, Hamburg

Evans RW (1992) Some observations on whiplash injuries. Neurol Clin 10:975–997

Fischer-Homberger E (1970) Railway spine and traumatic neuroses – the psyche and the spinal cord. Gesnerus 27:96–111

Freitag P, Greenlee MW, Wachter K, Ettlin TM, Radue EW (2001) fMRI response during visual motion stimulation in patients with late whiplash syndrome. Neurorehabil Neural Repair 15:31–37

Friberg L (1991) Cerebral blood flow changes in migraine. Methods, observations and hypotheses. J Neurol 238(Suppl 1):12–17

Friston KJ, Frith CD, Liddle PF, Frackowiak RSJ (1991) Comparing functional (PET) images: the assessment of significant change. J Cereb Blood Flow Metab 11:690–699

Friston KJ, Holmes AP, Worsley KJ, Poline JB, Frith CD, Frackowiak RSJ (1995a) Statistical parametric maps in functional imaging: a general approach. Hum Brain Mapp 2:189–210

Friston KJ, Ashburner J, Poline JB, Frith CD, Heather JD, Frackowiak RSJ (1995b) Spatial realignment and normalization of images. Hum Brain Mapp 2:165–189

Goethals I, Audenaert K, Jacobs F, Lannoo E, Van de Wiele C, Ham H, Otte A, Oostra K, Dierckx R (2004) Cognitive neuroactivation using SPECT and the Stroop colored word test in patients with diffuse brain injury. J Neurotrauma 21:1059–1069

Goldenberg G, Oder W, Spatt J, Podreka I (1992) Cerebral correlates of disturbed executive function and memory in survivors of severe closed head injury: a SPECT study. J Neurol Neurosurg Psychiatry 55:362–368

Graf M, Grill C, Wedig HD (eds) (2009) Beschleunigungsverletzung der Halswirbelsäule. Springer Steinkopff, Darmstadt

Graham DG, Brierly JB (1984) Vascular disorders of the central nervous system. In: Adams J (ed) Neuropathology. Edward Arnold, London, pp 125–207

Harrington R (1996) The 'railway spine' diagnosis and Victorian responses to PTSD. J Psychosom Res 40:11–14

Harwood DG, Barker WW, Loewenstein DA et al (1999) Cross-ethnic analysis of risk factors for AD in white Hispanics and white non-Hispanics. Neurology 52:551–556

Ichise M, Chung DG, Wang P, Wortzman G, Gray BG, Franks W (1994) Technetium-99m-HMPAO SPECT, CT and MRI in the evaluation of patients with chronic traumatic brain injury: a correlation with neuropsychological performance. J Nucl Med 35:217–226

Jacobs A, Put E, Ingels M, Bossuyt A (1994) Prospective evaluation of technetium-99m-HMPAO SPECT in mild and moderate traumatic brain injury. J Nucl Med 35:942–947

Johansson G, Risberg J, Rosenhall U, Orndahl G, Svennerholm L, Nystrom S (1995) Cerebral dysfunction in fibromyalgia: evidence from regional cerebral blood flow measurements, otoneurological tests and cerebrospinal fluid analysis. Acta Psychiatr Scand 91:86–94

Jörg J, Menger H (1998) Das Halswirbelsäulen- und Halsmarktrauma. Neurologische Diagnose und Differentialdiagnostik. Dtsch Ärztebl 95:B1048–B1055

Keller T (1995) Railway spine revisited: traumatic neurosis or neurotrauma? J Hist Med Allied Sci 50:507–524

Lass P, Lyczak P (2004) Functional neuroimaging in late whiplash syndrome and Alzheimer's disease. Hell J Nucl Med 7:58–59

Linnman C, Appel L, Söderlund A, Frans O, Engler H, Furmark T, Gordh T, Langström B, Frederikson M (2009) Chronic whiplash symptoms are related to altered regional cerebral blood flow in the resting state. Eur J Pain 13:65–70

Linnman C, Appel L, Furmark T, Soderlund A, Gordh T, Langstrom B, Fredrikson M (2010) Ventromedial prefrontal neurokinin 1 receptor availability is reduced in chronic pain. Pain 149:64–70

Linnman C, Appel L, Fredrikson M, Gordh T, Soderlund A, Langstrom B, Engler H (2011) Elevated [11 C]-D-deprenyl uptake in Chronic Whiplash Associated Disorder suggests persistent musculoskeletal inflammation. PLoS One 6:e19182. doi:10.1371/journal.pone. 001982

Linnman CN, Appel L, Furmark T, Söderlund A, Gordh T, Langström B, Fredrikson M (2012) Response to Dr. Otte: functional neuroimaging in whiplash injury. Eur J Pain 16(1):162–163

Liotti M, Mayberg HS (2001) The role of functional neuroimaging in the neuropsychology of depression. J Clin Exp Neuropsychol 23:121–136

Lorberboym M, Gilad R, Gorin V, Sadeh M, Lampl Y (2002) Late whiplash syndrome: correlation of brain SPECT with neuropsychological tests and P300 event-related potential. J Trauma 52:521–526

McConnell WE, Howard RP, Guzman HM et al (1993) Analysis of human test subject kinematic responses to low velocity rear end impacts. SAE Tech Paper Series 930889:21–30

McConnell WE, Howard RP, Poppel JV et al (1995) Human head and neck kinematic after low speed rear-end impacts: understanding "whiplash". 39th Stapp Car Crash Conference Proceedings 952724:215–238

Mehta KM, Ott A, Kalmijn S et al (1999) Head trauma and risk of dementia and Alzheimer's disease: the Rotterdam study. Neurology 52:1559–1562

Mesulam MM (1985) Principles of behavioural neurology. F.A. Davis, Philadelphia

Miller BL, Mena I, Daly J, Gombetti RJ, Goldberg MA, Lesser I, Garetti K, Villanueva-Meyer J, Liu CK (1990) Temporo-parietal hypoperfusion with single photon emission computerized tomography in conditions other than Alzheimer's disease. Dementia 1:41–45

Moskowitz MA, Buzzi MG (1991) Neuroeffector functions of sensory fibers. Implications for headache mechanisms and drug actions. J Neurol 238(Suppl 1):18–22

Olsson I, Bunketorp O, Carlsson G et al. (1990) An in-depth study of neck injuries in rear end car collisions. In: International IRCOBI conference, Bron, Lyon, 12–14 Sept 1990, pp 1–15

Ommaya AK, Faas F, Yarnell R (1968) Whiplash injury and brain damage: an experimental study. JAMA 204:75–79

Otte A (1998) Does whiplash trauma increase the risk of Alzheimer's disease? J Vasc Invest 4:211–212

Otte A (1999) PET with [18]fluorodexyglucose and hexamethylpropylene amine oxime SPECT in late whiplash syndrome. Neurology 52:1107–1108

Otte A (2000a) Kognitive Störungen nach traumatischer Distorsion der Halswirbelsäule: Schleudertrauma, quo vadis? Dtsch Ärztebl 97:A463

Otte A (2000c) The importance of the control group in functional brain imaging. Eur J Nucl Med 27:1420

Otte A (2000d) The parieto-occipital region – confusions at the boundary? Eur J Nucl Med 27:238–239

Otte A (2001a) The "railway spine" – a precursor for the "whiplash syndrome"? Med Sci Monit 7:1064–1065

Otte A (2001b) Eisenbahnkrankheit. Dtsch Ärztebl 98(34–35):A2173–A2174

Otte A (2001c) Das Halswirbelsäulen-Schleudertrauma: Neue Wege der funktionellen Bildgebung des Gehirns – Ein Ratgeber für Ärzte und Betroffene. Springer, Berlin, Heidelberg, New York, Tokyo

Otte A (2004) Functional neuroimaging in late whiplash syndrome and Alzheimer's disease. Hell J Nucl Med 7:59

Otte A (2012) Functional neuroimaging in whiplash injury. Eur J Pain 16(1):162–163. doi:10.1016/j.ejpain.2011.08.002

Otte A, Brändli M (1998) Olfactory distress following mild traumatic head injury: a SPECT follow-up. J Vasc Invest 4:207–209

Otte A, Halsband U (2006) Brain imaging tools in neuroimaging. J Physiol Paris 99:281–292

Otte A, Mueller-Brand J (1997) Is there a chronic fatigue of the late whiplash syndrome? J Vasc Invest 3:161

Otte A, Wink K (2008) Kerners Krankheiten großer Musiker. Die Neubearbeitung. 6., erw. Aufl., Schattauer, Stuttgart

Otte A, Ettlin TM, Mueller-Brand J (1995a) Comparison of Tc-99m-ECD with Tc-99m-HMPAO brain-SPECT in late whiplash syndrome. J Vasc Invest 1:157–163

Otte A, Mueller-Brand J, Fierz L (1995b) Brain SPECT findings in late whiplash syndrome. Lancet 345:1513–1514

Otte A, Ettlin Th, Fierz L, Mueller-Brand J (1996a) Parieto-occipital hypoperfusion in late whiplash syndrome: first quantitative SPET study using Tc-99m-bicisate (ECD). Eur J Nucl Med 23:72–74

Otte A, Ettlin TM, Fierz L, Kischka U, Muerner J, Högerle S, Bräutigam P, Mueller-Brand J (1996b) Zerebrale Befunde nach Halswirbelsäulendistorsion durch Beschleunigungsmechanismus (HWS-Schleudertrauma): Standortbestimmung zu neuen diagnostischen Methoden der Nuklearmedizin. [Cerebral findings after distorsion of the cervical spine induced by acceleration injury (whiplash injury): Assessment of current isotopic scanning techniques for diagnosis.]. Schweiz Rundsch Med Prax 85:1087–1090

Otte A, Ettlin TM, Fierz L, Kischka U, Muerner J, Mueller-Brand J (1997a) Brain perfusion patterns in 136 patients with chronic symptoms after distorsion of the cervical spine using single-photon emission computed tomography, technetium-99m-HMPAO and technetium-99m-ECD: a controlled study. J Vasc Invest 3:1–5

Otte A, Ettlin TM, Nitzsche EU, Wachter K, Hoegerle S, Simon GH, Fierz L, Moser E, Mueller-Brand J (1997b) PET and SPECT in whiplash syndrome: a new approach to a forgotten brain? J Neurol Neurosurg Psychiatry 63:368–372

Otte A, Ettlin TM, Otto I, Mueller-Brand J (1997c) Manipulation-triggered visual disturbances after cervical spine injury. J Vasc Invest 3:197–198

Otte A, Mueller-Brand J, Ettlin TM, Wachter K, Nitzsche EU (1997d) Functional imaging in 200 patients after whiplash injury. J Nucl Med 38:1002

Otte A, Weiner SM, Peter HH, Mueller-Brand J, Goetze M, Moser E, Gutfleisch J, Hoegerle S, Juengling FD, Nitzsche EU (1997e) Brain glucose utilization in systemic lupus erythematosus with beginning neuropsychiatric symptoms: a controlled PET study. Eur J Nucl Med 24:787–791

Otte A, Goetze M, Mueller-Brand J (1998a) Statistical parametric mapping in whiplash brain: is it only a contusion mechanism? Eur J Nucl Med 25:306–307

Otte A, Juengling FD, Nitzsche EU (1998b) Rethinking mild head injury. J Vasc Invest 4:45–46

Otte A, Stratz T, Wachter K, Nitzsche EU, Zajic T, Goetze M, Ettlin TM, Mueller-Brand J (1998c) Brain SPET Statistical Parametric Mapping (SPM) in fibromyalgia syndrome: Is brainstem perfusion impaired? J Vasc Invest 4:111–116

Otte A, Weiner SM, Hoegerle S, Wolf R, Juengling FD, Peter HH, Nitzsche EU (1998d) Neuropsychiatric systemic lupus erythematosus before and after immunosuppressive treatment: a FDG PET study. Lupus 7:57–59

Otte A, Audenaert K, Otte K (2003a) Did Maurice Ravel have a whiplash syndrome? Med Sci Monit 9:LE9

Otte A, de Bondt P, Van de Wiele C, Audenaert K, Dierckx RA (2003b) The exceptional brain of Maurice Ravel. Med Sci Monit 9:RA154–RA159

Poeck K (1999) Kognitive Störungen nach traumatischer Distorsion der Halswirbelsäule? Dtsch Ärztebl 96:A2596–A2601

Radanov BP, Bicik I, Dvorak J, Antinnes J, von Schulthess GK, Buck A (1999) Relation between neuropsychological and neuroimaging findings in patients with late whiplash syndrome. J Neurol Neurosurg Psychiatry 66:485–489

Ryan GA, Taylor GW, Moore V, Dolinis J (1993) Neck strain in car occupants. Med J Aust 159:651–656

Schmid P (1999) Whiplash-associated disorders. Schweiz Med Wochenschr 25:1368–1380

Severy DM, Mathewson JH, Bechtol CO (1955) Controlled automobile rear-end collisions, an investigation of related engineering and mechanical phenomenon. Can Services Med J 11:727–758

Spitzer WO, Skovron ML, Salmi LR et al (1995) Quebec Task Force on Whiplash-Associated Disorders: scientific monographs of the Quebec Task Force on Whiplash-Associated Disorders. Redefining "whiplash" and its management. Spine 20(Suppl):1–73

Sundström T, Guez M, Hildingsson C, Toolanen G, Nyberg L, Riklund K (2006) Altered cerebral blood flow in chronic neck pain patients but not in whiplash patients: a ^{99m}Tc-HMPAO rVBF study. Eur Spine J 15:1189–1195

Talairach J, Tournoux P (1988) Co-planar atlas of the human brain. Georg Thieme Verlag, Stuttgart, New York

Talairach J, Tournoux P (1993) Referentially oriented cerebral MRI anatomy. Atlas of stereotaxic anatomical correlations for gray and white matter. Georg Thieme Verlag, Stuttgart, New York

Tashiro M, Juengling F, Reinhardt M, Moser E, Nitzsche E (2000) Psychological response and survival in breast cancer. Lancet 355:405–406

Thompson RS, Rivara FP, Thompson DC (1989) A case–control study of the effectiveness of bicycle safety helmets. N Engl J Med 320:1361–1367

Waldemar G, Bruhn P, Kristensen M, Johnsen A, Paulson O, Lassen NA (1994) Heterogeneity of neocortical cerebral blood flow deficits in dementia of the Alzheimer Type: a ^{99m}Tc-HMPAO-SPECT study. J Neurol Neurosurg Psychiatry 57:285–295

Weiner SM, Otte A (2004) Neuropsychiatric involvement in systemic lupus erythematosus. In: Otte A, Audenaert K, Peremans K, Van Heering C, Dierckx RA (eds) Nuclear medicine in psychiatry. Springer, Berlin, Heidelberg, New York, Hong Kong, London, Milan, Paris, Tokyo, pp 233–271

Weiner SM, Otte A, Schumacher M, Klein R, Gutfleisch J, Otto P, Brink I, Nitzsche EU, Moser E, Peter HH (2000) Diagnosis and monitoring of central nervous system involvement in systemic lupus erythematosus: value of F-18 fluorodeoxyglucose PET. Ann Rheum Dis 59:377–385

West DH, Gough JP, Harper TK (1993) Low speed collision testing using human subjects. Accid Reconstr J 5:22–26

Index